The More You Explain The Less They Understand

Ruth Velikovsky Sharon, Ph.D.
and
John Cathro Seed, M.D.

Illustrations: Ralph Schlegel

Paradigma

Internet: www.ruthvelikovskysharon.com
e-mail: ruthvsharonphd@verizon.net

Drawings: Ralph Schlegel
Cover illustration: Ralph Schlegel

Published by Paradigma Ltd.
Internet: www.paradigma-publishing.com
e-mail: info@paradigma-publishing.com

ISBN 978-1-906833-00-8

Contents

Acknowledgements

Rafael Sharon for his valuable contribution.

This book would not have been possible without the intensive help of David Nagel.

Ralph Schlegel contributed the art. His talent and awareness of the human condition are unsurpassed.

Benjamin Cittadino whose knowledge, advice and integrity are unmatched in his field.

Catherine Karpowicz for her pleasant competence.

Mark Janus for his reliability and expertise.

Richard Peterson for help with the euphemisms.

John O'Donnell for his consistent good advice.

Carmel Warner for her competent approach to education.

Naomi Mitchell for her creativity.

Introduction

Many loving parents mistakenly believe that by bestowing their children with everything – by granting their every wish, and pleasing their every whim – they are outperforming as parents, when in fact – the opposite is true. "No" represents authority, giving the parents control and empowerment. As one mother summed it: "I am a good mother because I won't let my children get away with any nonsense and I am involved in their education, making certain they are prepared for life."

Parents whose children grow up respecting their physical health, not overeating, not abusing alcohol and not smoking, have done a good job raising them! In addition, making certain their children get the best education is a priority. Not overindulging their children, while disciplining them will help accomplish all of the above.

Overindulgent parents rationalize their child rearing, thinking that if they adore their children and repeatedly reward them, the children will grow up to be successful adults. This approach more often yields the opposite result.

Parents whose attitude is: "My children are grown now, so they are responsible for their own behavior and actions" should be asked, at what point should parents toss aside their responsibility for the way their grown offspring turned out? The answer, which parents don't want to accept, is: "Never!"

Two teenagers kicked a homeless man to death, because "it was something to do" and "it was fun." If the parents of these teenagers are alive, they, as well as the teenagers, should be held legally accountable for the crime. Standing in court and crying for their children who are about to be sentenced to jail is letting parents off too easy! Once parents fear that the consequences of overindulging their children will be put squarely and legally on their shoulders, refraining from overindulging their children will take on a new meaning. Had they disciplined their children, taught them right from wrong and not overindulged them, while providing them with the best education, the result could have been law-abiding adults successful in career and in marriage.

I
Daddy's Girl

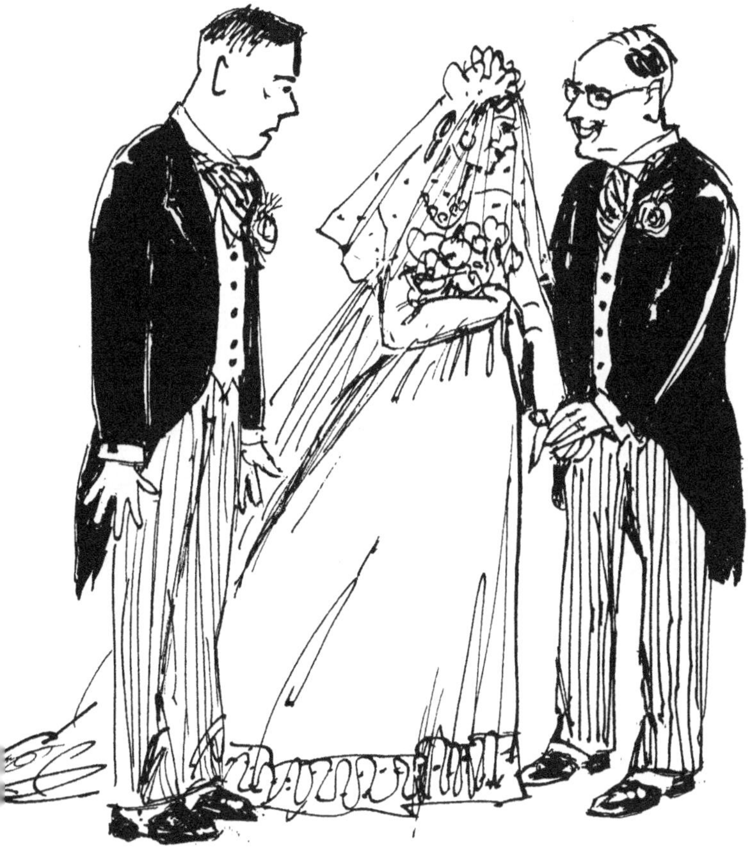

Daddy's Girl

The little girl who is adored by her father grows up convinced that her husband is supposed to adore her the way her father did. Having repeatedly been told that she is wonderful, exceptional, special, she grows up expecting her husband to admire everything about her! When these expectations are not met, inconsistency between her husband's perception and her self-perception creates conflict, first within her, then in their relationship. Her receptors don't receive the right information to validate her narcissism. The slightest, most trivial incident might upset her. Behavioral patterns between the two inevitably develop; a continuous tightening and loosening of the line between them that is the notion of her "specialness", leading her to anger, depression and withdrawal.

If the man who marries a Daddy's Girl does not fulfill her expectations (which he won't) she will admonish him: "You didn't even kiss me good-morning" and remind him: "Aren't you proud of me for the meal I prepared?" She complains to others: "He doesn't look at me. He doesn't say good-morning. He literally shuts off. He treats me like a leper. What? Because the room is messy? Everything has to be his way. What have I done that is so terrible? It can't be his way or the highway!" If she doesn't get her way, she shuts down, which is no different than what a three year old does lying down in the middle of a store kicking and screaming. Basically her attitude is: "I am me; I'm supposed to be adored merely because of the qualities I possess: my looks, my personality, everything about me." In therapy, if the couple seeks professional marital conflict resolution, she is unable to look at herself through any other lens. If the therapist suggests that she might adjust in a certain way, her immediate response is: "What about <u>him</u>?" (There's nothing wrong with me!). It's inconceivable to her that she might be part of, or the reason for their problem.

When her husband is apologetic, she then launches into more recriminating attacks. She sounds like an actress playing deaf as she proceeds to vomit a crescendo of feelings. Daddy's Girl plays the "game" her father encouraged: She is wonderful and beyond! She is entitled and deserving! When asked "What are you doing wrong?" she replies: "I am not perfect, I'm not the neatest person in the world. No. Until our marriage he took me out, spent time with me. He married me – then he dropped me like a hot potato. How was I supposed to know – that the minute he put the ring on my finger, that I am going to be a prop. What on earth justifies treating me like this! He is uncommunicative and I am totally emotionally deprived."

The irony is that Daddy's Girl will likely marry a difficult, yet educated, successful, outspoken and critical man. She argues while not hearing what her husband says. She is tuned to a different channel – the one that proclaims she is right! When her husband points out to her how she might improve, she punches back verbally!
Daddy's Girl treats her children in a similar way to the way she was treated growing up. She will interfere with her husband's disciplining the children, saying: "They are tired," "They are hungry," and supervising him: "Leave them alone," causing her own children to be overgratified. The mother is the boss in raising the children – while her husband acquiesces, or there is war! And, finally, Grandpa, the originator of the problem, re-enters the picture and "honeys" the grandchildren.

The father who paints his daughter's image on the canvas of life enwrapped in diamonds – sends the message: "She is perfect" and that the mother is being replaced. Father-daughter dances held at community centers send out a perverse message. Why haven't they sponsored mother-son dances? Why does that sound unacceptable and father-daughter dances are considered O.K.?

Daddy's Girl is often hypochondriacal and suffers from disease de jour (illness of the day). A couple of years into the marriage Daddy's Girl lets herself go, gaining weight and looking unappealing, yet her husband is supposed to adore her! She smokes and drinks, as her husband loses his sexual feelings for her and tells her that he could go without sex and without talking to her for months, that she is totally inferior to him and that he fell for the act and married her – only to be the sole person on earth to soon find out who she really was! Contrary to Daddy's Girl's expectations, her husband, instead of reading the "cue-cards" of adoration she prepared for him, he tells her unedited negative comments of what he really thinks, that she is the only one who doesn't listen to him, and that their marriage is permanently unfulfilling to him as well as boring and that he feels stuck! He then adds that a smart person knows there are smarter people than them, and his wife doesn't recognize that he is smarter than she is and that since her parents were not terribly bright, it's a double whammy, for at least other married women are imbued with skills that she isn't. He then says that he comes up for air only to bang his head against the wall. He has to keep his mind submerged or he becomes overwhelmed by the truth flooding in.

Daddy's Girl's problem is not that she doesn't hear or listen, it is that she doesn't digest. She takes everything her husband says superficially and at face value. Repeatedly told by her daddy that she was special, set her up for a lifetime of "because Daddy said so". She has no idea what she is not good at, and insists on having an opinion about areas that she doesn't have a clue about. She won't admit she doesn't know what it's about because Daddy told her she is the best. Her husband becomes angry at her for being impervious to her limitations. He can't get it through to her to understand that she got as far as she did only because of her people pleasing skills.

Daddy's Girl will complain that she is exhausted from dealing with her husband and that their relationship deteriorates day by day. She sulks and mopes while her husband distances himself to escape the misery. Having been accustomed to being told by her father how wonderful she is, she accuses her husband of not appreciating her, and in fact, undermining her and mistreating her. Blinded to the role she plays, she claims innocence and that she can do no wrong, as she fools the world with her deceptive presentation.

The father who creates the perfect female in his life – his daughter – whom he adores from day one, unintentionally ruins her life! Meaning well, thinking that if he lavishes on her constant affection, toys, vacations and attention, that when she grows up she will have had an example of what an adoring male should be like and she will thus know what she wants in a husband! However, no matter who she marries, if she marries at all, she will have expectations her husband will not be able to meet. Daddy's Girl will soon feel neglected, pleading with her husband to throw her a bone, to give her some respect and companionship so she doesn't feel that he is condescending and dismissive. She badmouths him to her children and to her friends, harming his reputation with lies and exaggerations. She wants her husband to recognize her brilliance instead of finishing her sentences, which she finds exceedingly infantilizing. When criticized, she withdraws into a cocoon. She claims that her love for her husband is a waste of her time since he is dehumanizing because he never understood what she gave him. As a result she sulks under the covers of narcissistic injury, while her husband is relentlessly critical, complaining that "she is a piece of work". He then hibernates in his room for hours at a time, bemoaning his fate of being married to a controlling actress. He wants to come and go as he pleases, while thinking: "I'm like a scared little rabbit: A man afraid of his wife". While calling his wife handicapped and a burden – she nevertheless sees herself as an asset who can never please him! Whenever he talks to her he feels as though he is talking to his teacher, for she admonishes him for wanting the freedom to think for himself!

When a woman says her father was her best friend, she either remains single, never finding the "perfect" mate, or she enters an unrewarding marriage. The man who is about to ask for her hand in marriage should be cautioned. Growing up, she seemed to have everything, for it was her father's delight to grant her every whim. How would the script her father was playing equip her for the realities of adult life, love and marriage? What would happen when Daddy's Girl left the safe and overprotective home her father had created for her? He thought: "I'll adore her and do everything for her and she will grow up a successful adult and have a good life." Well, surprise, surprise, it works in reverse. The overindulgent father destroys his daughter's emotional muscles, while growing into an adult with unreasonable expectations, who will have a "Daddy" script and symbolic cue cards for her husband to recite.

Little does the father know that by repeatedly telling his daughter: "All I want for you is to be happy in life," he is giving her an impossible assignment, since happiness is elusive, and, at best, intermittent. His ill-advised overindulgence hinders her from settling down with one partner and from becoming a financially responsible contributing partner, causing her to flounder from profession to profession, looking for the one that will make her happy. It is an unachievable assignment, likely to set her up for a life sentence of unhappiness.

The father who worships his daughter, never raising his voice, saying only adoring words to her day in and day out, causes her, as she grows to adulthood, to have unreasonable expectations of her husband. Not aware of the dangers of his overindulgence, the father works hard to make his little girl feel special. He eventually sees warnings that his favorite child will grow up to become ill equipped to take care of herself and that his overindulgence will program her to become a parasite, needing a host to leech onto. Nevertheless, believing his beloved daughter will become secure in the charms he had taught her to value, thriving on her ability to prompt adoration, she becomes a fake and only her husband knows who she really is.

The father who favors his daughter and makes her number one, complicates the mother/daughter relationship, the mother resenting both the father and the daughter. The mother/daughter incompatibility, often erupting during the girl's teens, is heightened by competition for the one man. The father, if over-solicitous, particularly if physically demonstrative to his daughter, will prevent the natural resolution of the problem, while the mother, feeling neglected, will resent her daughter, who in turn, will feel threatened by the role she is permitted to play in her parents' lives.

One father complimented his grown daughter bragging out loud to those within earshot: "Did you hear how she handled that phone call? Wow! She is unbelievable! What talent! What expertise!" Daddy's Girl's husband is not impressed with her phone conversations as her father still is, nor any other conversations for that matter she has with anyone, nor her people pleasing skills, as he thinks to himself: "When our kids are grown and leave, what am I going to talk to my wife about? She just wants compliments!"

Once his wife goes to bed he calms his frustrations by going into the kitchen to stuff his face. Having given up alcohol and drugs he becomes a food addict. Once he crawls into bed, she wakes up and turns to him and asks: "Don't you think I look good?" His answer, which he withholds, is "No". He is at his wit's end while she feels she is getting nothing from him, and that he is non-communicative. She tells him: "I just get to a point where I feel I've had it!" That makes her husband want to celebrate: "It's over!" But it's not!

To complicate matters, the wife uses the grown children as weapons to keep her husband in line and monitor him, while she reads his e-mails and checks his car nightly. His children assume the job of "parenting" their father and ridiculing him for wanting out of the marriage. He describes his wife as wanting to be complimented, but without basis. While she confides in the children, she gives them the unspoken assignment of "straightening" out their father.

If the mother/daughter relationship is fraught with rejection, the daughter, as she grows up, may seek the "good breast" in a relationship with another woman.

Parents and their offspring have their assigned roles. They are not friends nor pals. When the children take over the parental role, it is loaded with potential trouble for all concerned. By being his child's friend the parent deprives the child of normal outside relationships. What the parent imparts about himself is that he lacks a good relationship with the spouse and hence needs a close emotional tie with his offspring. This burden places an unnatural responsibility on the offspring. A parent who complains to his child about the other parent while implying that it's to be kept a secret, creates emotional stress for his child. No matter how old the child and what the parent's complaint is, the child should not be the parent's confidant.

One Daddy's Girl who had been allowed to rule the family, wouldn't let anyone film her tenth birthday party. Nobody dared. For no apparent reason she stopped dead in her tracks. "I don't want my brother here! I am not going to let anyone have cake until he leaves!" Father whispered to Tommy to slide out of the room on cue. "Now you switch seats and you sit here, and you sit there," she instructed her subjects. Among her most willing was her father, who took delight in his daughter's brattyness. The ten year old had free rein and dictatorship, where she held everyone in her family hostage.

Children whose birthdays are celebrated ad nauseum will grow up expecting the spouse to carry on the tradition. A Daddy's Girl arranged a luncheon celebration for her fortieth birthday, saying she was not going to wait for her husband to do something nice for her on her birthday, so she is going to throw herself a "little" party with her best friends. She considered it fun, and it would make her feel good! She excluded her husband – he wasn't invited. Having bad-mouthed him to her friends, they were not surprised that he wasn't going to attend the party. She told her husband that she never said negative things about him to her friends – which comes under the heading of deception – a typical Daddy's Girl maneuver.

One Daddy's Girl enjoyed being adored and admired, while her younger sister, an unplanned child, was an "inconvenience", the father repeatedly spanking her throughout her life. As he aged, the father sank into depressions and was hospitalized several times, the younger daughter was by his side. The mother who appreciated her younger daughter's devotion and care of her father, wrote about it in a number of handwritten pages. The older daughter (the Daddy's Girl) hid these pages from her sister, and never returned them.

II
Mommy's Boy

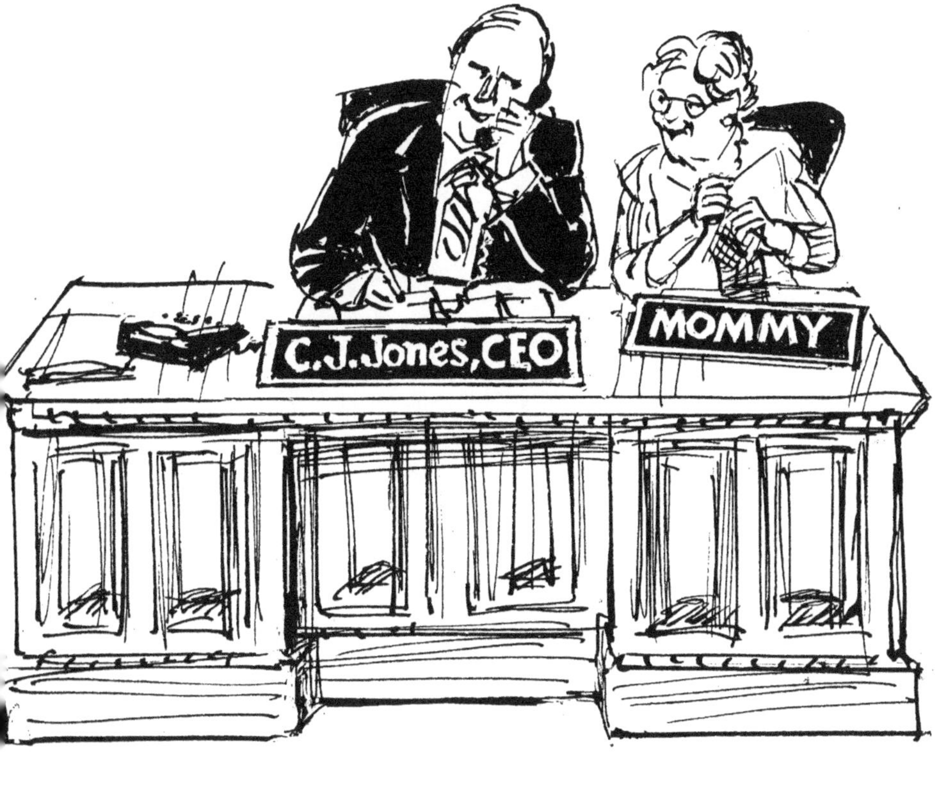

Mommy's Boy

The mother who bestows unrestrained adoration on her son with whom she cuddles while being touchy feely, is destructive beyond repair. Lavishing frequent physical affection on her son will cause him to grow up confused about his sexuality. Believing her son will grow up to love women because he loves her so much, she will find quite the opposite. Not only that, the son's relationship to the father deteriorates when the mother adores the son more than she adores her husband, and the son eventually earns his father's resentment, and as a result, the son leaves all women to the father to "stay out of trouble."

It is detrimental when a mother carries her son physically and emotionally much too close, forming a bond that sequesters him from peers and an upbringing with normalcy for young boys. This is especially troubling when he is distanced from the role model normally provided by Daddy, because of the exaggerated sense of the mother's love and protection. Without the proper male role model, he is likely to run into stumbling blocks during adolescent development, i.e. his interest in girls, participation in sports, and other social bonding that boys do together, while running the risk of the confusion taking the form of bi-sexuality.

The mother who, when her son reaches puberty, still has her arm around him, demonstrating in public how loving she is and what a "wonderful" mother she is, is destructive. Being unaware that her cuddly, lovey, touchy, feely adoration sent him on a difficult path of homosexuality he will remember his relationship to his mother as wonderful and that she did no wrong. Throughout adulthood this man will speak highly of his mother – that she really understood him and adored him. He will likely confide in her his sexual experiences, while excluding his father from his confidence. In fact, the father may not find out, and only suspect, that his son is gay!

Answering an ad for an assistant, a young man was hired to organize the archives of a famous person. Having been adored by his mother, (his father unaware that he was gay), he felt entitled and began stealing some of the archives. His deceptive presentation got him hired, only to be fired once valuable papers were missing and some of the author's out of print books appeared on Amazon.com with the young man's name as the seller. Being related to a person in the legal field, he was advised and protected from getting into legal trouble. His mother, who overindulged him, created three fundamental lifetime problems for him: one, homosexuality, the second dishonesty and the third a poor and almost non-existent relationship with his father. The mother was in charge – her son confiding in her (as well as in the person who hired him) his first sexual contact with a male. The physical, huggy kissy adoration created homosexuality and "Whatever makes you happy" resulted in dishonesty.

When asked about his upbringing, the homosexual male will typically recall having seen his mother in a state of partial or complete undress (a screen memory – one experience symbolizing many) arousing his curiosity and physical sensations he did not understand at the time. The mother who consciously tries to become THE woman in her son's life, will cause him, when he grows up, to remain "loyal" to her, and no other woman will be physically or psychologically appealing to him. As he grows up, if he gets married, he may have difficulty relating sexually to his wife. On an unconscious level he may experience having sex with his wife as a betrayal of his mother, thereby causing impotence. In addition, the father's resentment of his wife's and son's closeness will cast fear in the son. A mother who relates to her adult son as her friend and confidant, sharing late night hugs and conversations, compromises her son's sexuality. The father, relegated to an observer, no longer has any effect on his adult son's sexual identity, while the mother feels innocent, not realizing the ingredient she was introducing into her son's life which had a profound effect.

One boy, physically pampered by an adoring mother, when grown up, ventured into adulthood suffering from a sexual perversion. Exposing himself to housekeepers, who fulfilled his seemingly innocent request to bring him a towel to the bathroom door, where he stood naked, his penis erect, as he uttered: "Don't be afraid!" Since exhibitionism and voyeurism go hand in hand, he also spent hours peering from behind his window curtain into another window, hoping to see a woman undressing.

Mommy's Boy does not take the form of a latent experience affecting only sexuality. Young boys grow up not knowing how to do for themselves what their mothers gorged them within their care and provision. When it comes time to leave the nest, they never quite make the leap. The mother clings to the relationship, which says it all on Mother's Day, when she looks at the calendar wondering if her boy will send her a card! Mother's Day is a holiday for the "insulted" mother to savor every moment of neglect!

One mother started the tradition of giving her one year old a bedtime hug. At the age of two she gave him two hugs. At the age of three – three hugs. How long was that to continue?

One father complained to his wife his frustrations of the way she brought up their son, who was a playboy and an aggravation to his parents. He got into trouble by punching someone, cursing someone or crashing his car, while never earning a penny, which did not bother him. The father, having reached the end of his rope, called him an adult infant while the mother, who did not feel responsible for her son's problems, continued to do his laundry, cook for him and feed him.

The mother who insists on being her son's best friend through all his years of development, hampers his making his own friends. It is not natural for a boy growing into his teens, to prefer the company of his mother to his peers. At a certain age every healthy teenager will break away from emotional and physical dependency on his parents. If that break never comes, the teenager will walk through life with emotional crutches.

One mother told her grown son that they were husband and wife in a former life.

The father and son competition will resolve itself providing the mother does not interfere on behalf of the boy. One mother complained that her husband insists on admonishing and instructing their son at the "wrong time", when the boy is barely able to keep his eyes open. What is most damaging for the boy, however, was sensing that his mother sympathized with him, thereby undermining his relationship to his father.

A woman, loving her son more than her husband, invariably damages all three. The relationship between parents – imparting a solid marriage – helps the child understand his role in the family and, later on in life, he will select a mate who has the positive traits of both parents. Parents who are miserable with each other, while expressing exaggerated affection for their child, confiding in him private problems, will stand in the way of his normal sexual adjustment.

III
Overgratification

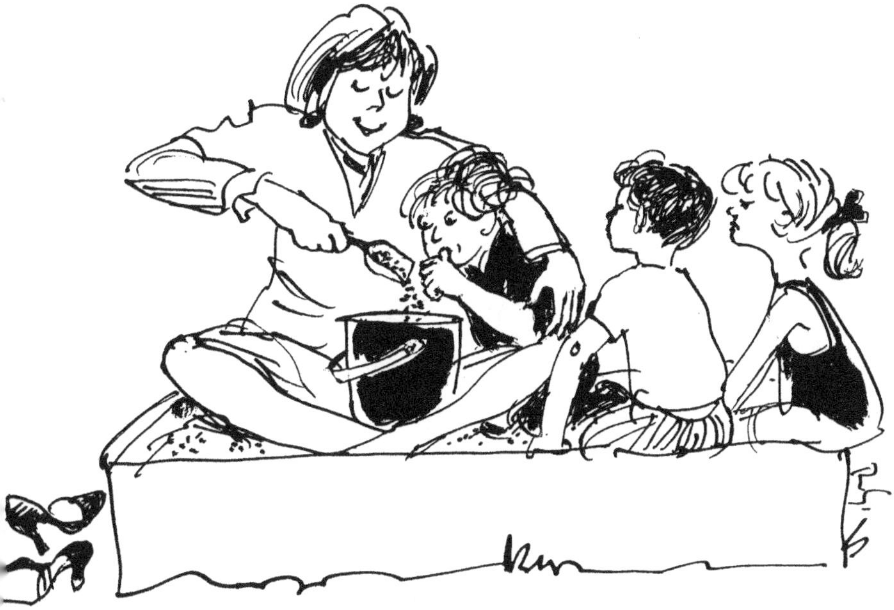

You are SPECIAL ... You are SPECIAL ... You are SPECIAL!

Overgratification

Parents most often overindulge their first-born, announcing: "I've created this wonderful baby and I'll do everything to make him happy 100% of the time and he will grow up to be a big success!" Unfortunately it is likely that he will grow into a non-functioning narcissist sequestered in his room wanting to be loved, unable to cope with the frustrations of life, expecting his family to orbit around his every whim. Excessively sensitive, the narcissist, who is difficult to love, requires gentle care. Mental hospitals are full of people who have been overindulged and not overfrustrated, as is a common belief.

A balance of frustration and gratification when raising children is essential for their healthy development. While it is better to err on the side of frustration rather than gratification, physical punishment is inadvisable, while gratification does not include: "O.K., O.K., you can have whatever you want". Many adults wish, in retrospect, that they had had parents who pushed them to learn and develop their talents! One father had his twelve year old play the cello, learn French, Spanish, Latin, Fencing, Tai Kwon-Do and the list goes on, all expressing the father's caring!

One misbehaved six year old's grandmother told him: "You are a brat!" to which he replied: "No, I'm not!" which says it all. Only a brat would respond: "I'm not!" as though he knows better than the grandmother. A child who is not a brat would not have responded, or would have inquired: "What did I do?"
When the grandmother said to her eight year old grandson: "I'm the wicked witch!" he replied: "You are not the wicked witch – you are a strict witch!" showing understanding and promise.

Growing up, the overindulged child will identify with the negative qualities of each parent, while the disciplined child will identify with the positive qualities of each parent. The parent who was himself overgratified, will perpetuate the problem and raise overgratified children, the problem continuing from generation to generation.

People throughout their lives will induce in others the predominant feeling their parents had for them. The phenomenon of the parents' feelings and treatment "bouncing" off the child, reveals how the child was brought up, which will last a lifetime. The child who was frequently spanked, once grown, will become a host to a parasite inducing in others the desire to mistreat him physically. The overindulged child will pretend to be sweet, as the parent "instructed", thereby collecting adoration from the outside world (but not from the spouse who sees the act). A child whose parents cared enough to discipline him, while vigilantly monitoring his intellectual and physical development, will grow up respectful of others, while at the same time being respectful of himself.

The child repeatedly told he was "special", and that he will do great things in life, will become obsessed with wanting, and actually expecting, to have his name in lights, receiving applause he was accustomed to receive from his parents. If unable to achieve notoriety, he will become jealous of the successful and will, as an antidote, try to make them jealous of him, by marrying a celebrity, owning designer clothes, a big house, an expensive car, etc. If that does not make others jealous of him, he will become vindictive and "push down" those who keep him from achieving his goal, subjecting them to rejection, eventually cutting them off completely.

Children who were rarely disciplined, where rules and boundaries were disregarded, then when on rare occasions they were told to clean their room or do their homework, when grown they may recall such occurrences as ongoing monumental abuse their entire childhood. As they grow up, these children will bad-mouth their parents, saying they were abused, abusing the word "abuse" their entire life.

Parents who mistakenly use questions, such as: "When are you going to stop fighting?" or "Why haven't you cleaned your room?" are not soliciting answers. Parents who add "O.K.?" when instructing their child, weaken the command, while saying "thank you" to a child who obeys the parent, undermines the parent. Obedience should be expected. When a parent, as a disciplinary act, tells his child to go to his room for an assigned period of time, and the child refuses to obey, he is taken by the hand and led to his room. Reprieve for good behavior, such as: "When you stop crying you can come out," puts the child in command and defeats the purpose of discipline.

A 10 year old girl was told by her father: "Either you sit down like a nice girl, or you are going to get time out," to which she replied: "You can't give me time out because I'm not going in my room!" "I'll put you in the guest room," responded the father, to which the girl said: "There are no lights in there." This type of back and forth discussion is tantamount to giving the child control. Rather than arguing back and forth, where the child tries to persuade the parent to "give me another chance", the parent must be in charge at all times The more you explain, the less they understand. Explanations too often give the child the opportunity to argue and disobey.

Parents who themselves were overindulged, too often perpetuate the problem. Being unaware of the dangers overindulgence hoisted upon their children manifests, these parents play out scripts from their own emotional scarring that life had brought them. Punishment meted out to train a child to know right from wrong – and not stemming from the parent's tensions of a hard day's work, is parental responsibility.

Afraid of hurting the "fragile little creature", parents use qualifiers which unravel their instructions, inviting the child to disagree, disobey and argue.

Some qualifiers:

Essentially, usually, often, ordinarily, perchance, perhaps, hopefully, possibly, preferably, presumably, probably, seems to, should, someday, somehow, sometimes, sort of, sounds like, the truth is, to a degree, unless, until, whatever, whenever, apparently, at times, attempt, consider, contemplate, eventually, frequently, generally speaking, happen to, I anticipate, I believe, I could, I guess, I imagine, I may, I might, I think, I would, I'll try, if, in time, kind of, likely, maybe, more often than not, most of the time, not infrequently, not necessarily, now and then, occasionally, ponder, my goal.

A child treated as though he is fragile and talked to only in loving tones, while keeping all noise away, will be unaccustomed to hearing anything unpleasant and, as he grows up, will emotionally collapse when subjected to the slightest frustration that life has in store. Convinced that to overlook their children's every little accomplishment is neglectful, parents don't realize that the child will attain more, as he grows up, if his minor accomplishments are not fussed over. Parents who use glowing adjectives to describe their children's accomplishments, whether within the children's earshot, are not doing their children a service! Displaying posters praising the child with such adjectives as: enchanting, outstanding, astonishing, astounding, shocking, extraordinary, phenomenal, do the child more harm than good. The child who is repeatedly told he is "special" will hold up symbolic "cue cards" instructing his family to meet his expectations. Unable to survive except in a womb-like environment, the tasks of life being too difficult, the child will become a lifelong parasite, frantically searching for a host to take care of him.

Children's degree of intelligence (I.Q.) depends on their genes, as does their appearance (height, eye color, etc.), but their behavior is greatly dependent on the way they were raised. A disciplined child will become a responsible hard working adult, knowing the boundaries between truths and lies and between mine and yours. The overindulged child will disregard boundaries thinking: "I can take what I want, and do what I want because I am special. I was never punished for anything." The disciplined child grows up a lot more responsible than the child who is repeatedly told "you're adorable, you're wonderful, you're superb. Do whatever will make you happy."

An overgratified two year old, who is given a bottle when he can and wants to drink from a glass, who is carried when he is able to walk, gets the message that to grow up and fend for himself is undesirable. The child constantly admired and fussed over may grow up self-conscious, as though he is in his own movie observing himself on camera. Parents who tell their child that he is a genius will cause him to live outside reality, where a gap will exist between his belief that he is a genius and his poor functioning.

Making decisions involves assuming responsibility and facing consequences. The natural process of life demands that a young person become independent, and independence means thinking and doing for himself! A good rule for parents to abide by is: Don't do for the child what he can do for himself. He will thus, at every stage of development, discard the words "I can't" or "help me". This rule sets the direction for an eventual independence, acquired slowly, which is far less painful to both parent and child than independence gained in a harsh break in the later teen years, when the teenager is not accustomed to test his independence.

Respect for time measures a person's emotional health: always late – hostile; always early – anxious; setting the clock ahead to fool himself into being on time – emotionally unstable! The person who stays up half the night and then can't get up in the morning was overindulged as a child. The perfectionist blames lack of time for leaving tasks undone. The emotionally healthy person tends to responsibilities, respecting his own mortality. Tardiness which inflicts anxiety on close family members who imagine an infinite number of calamities, could be spared the anguish in this day of the cell phone. In addition, the tardy person will react negatively to nagging ("go already!"), and blame the nagger for delaying him.

The Brat and The Good Child

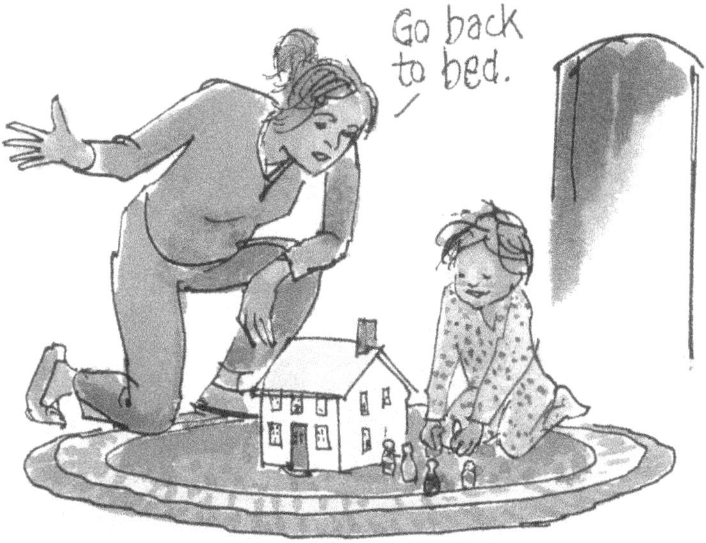
Go back to bed.

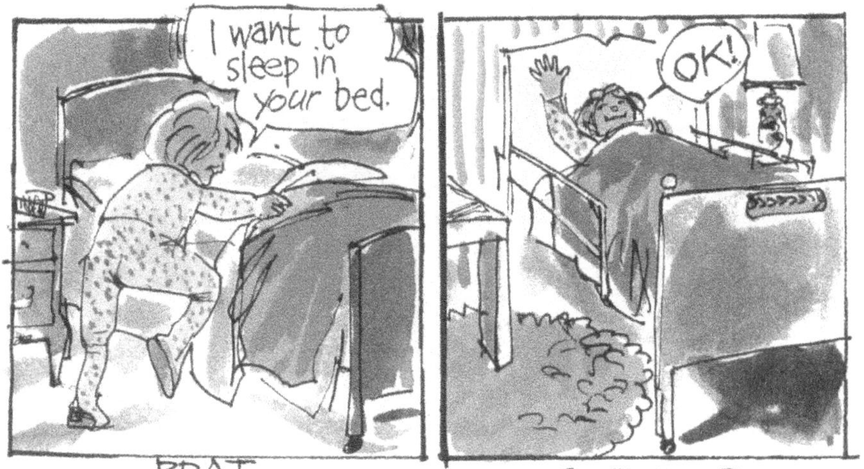
I want to sleep in your bed.
OK!

BRAT GOOD CHILD

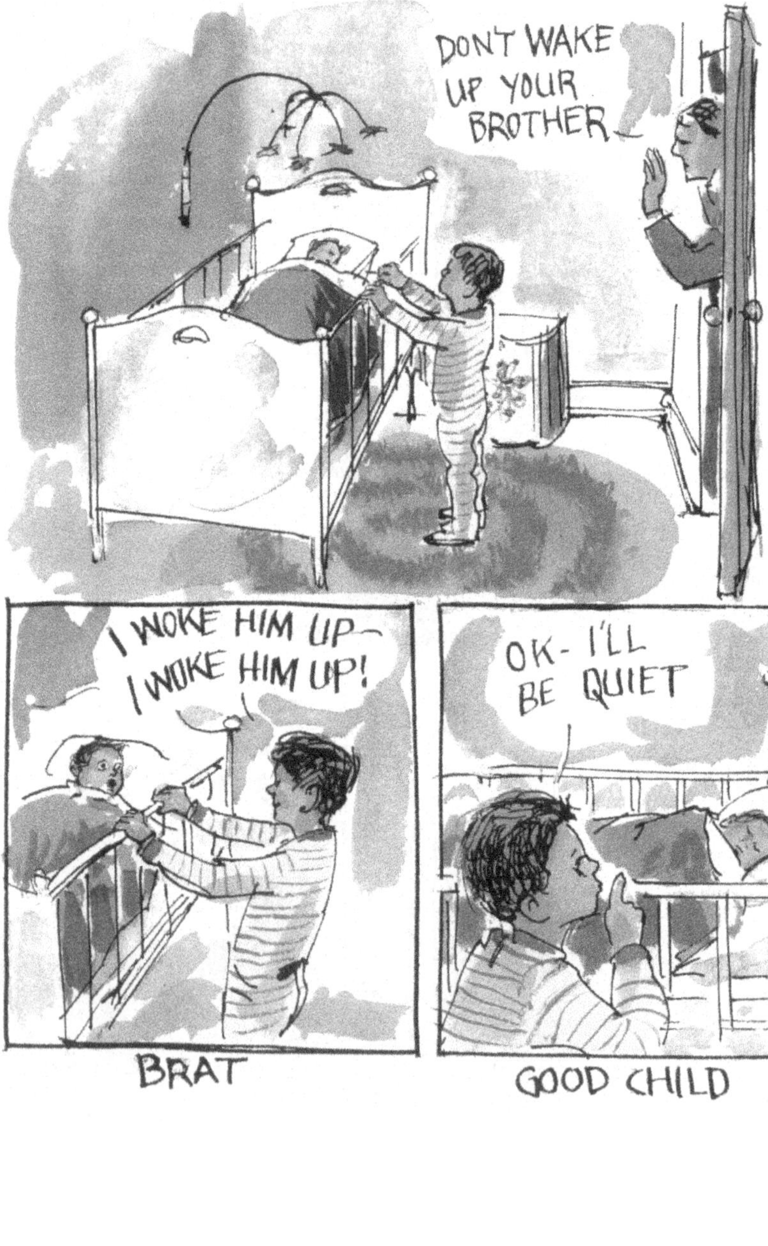
DON'T WAKE UP YOUR BROTHER
I WOKE HIM UP— I WOKE HIM UP!
BRAT
OK- I'LL BE QUIET
GOOD CHILD

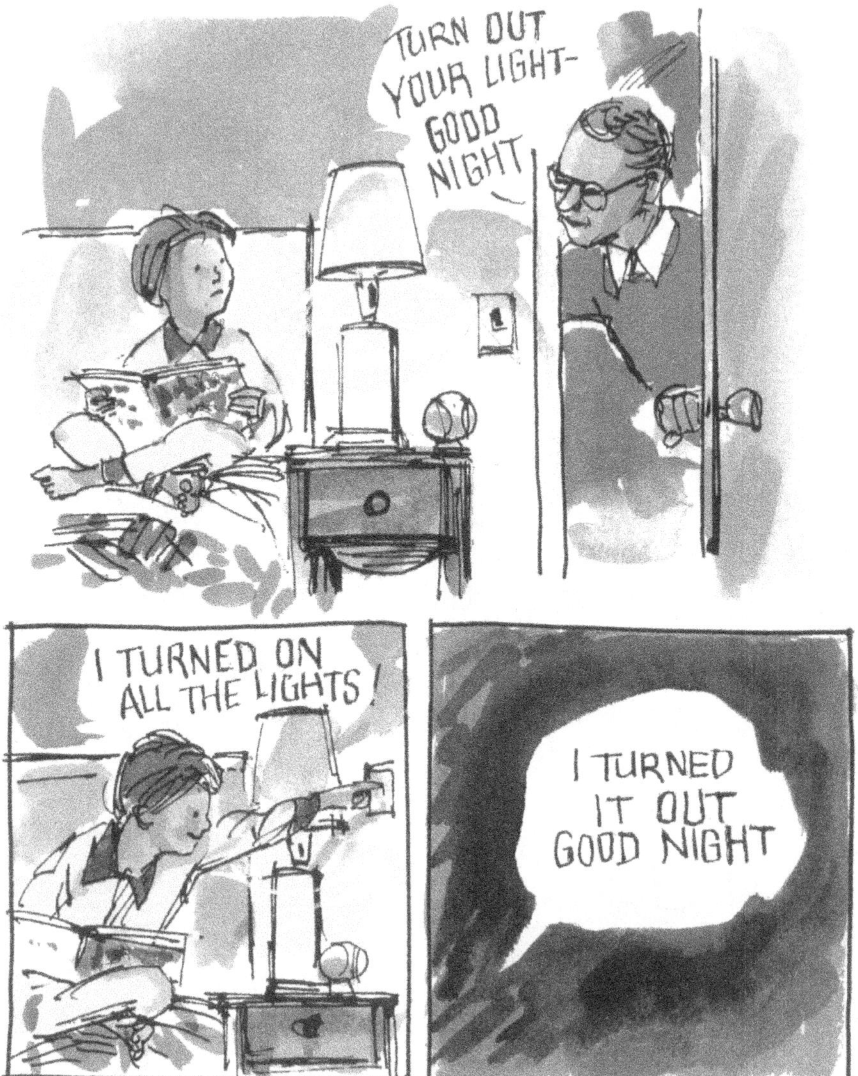
TURN OUT YOUR LIGHT- GOOD NIGHT
I TURNED ON ALL THE LIGHTS!
BRAT
I TURNED IT OUT GOOD NIGHT
GOOD CHILD

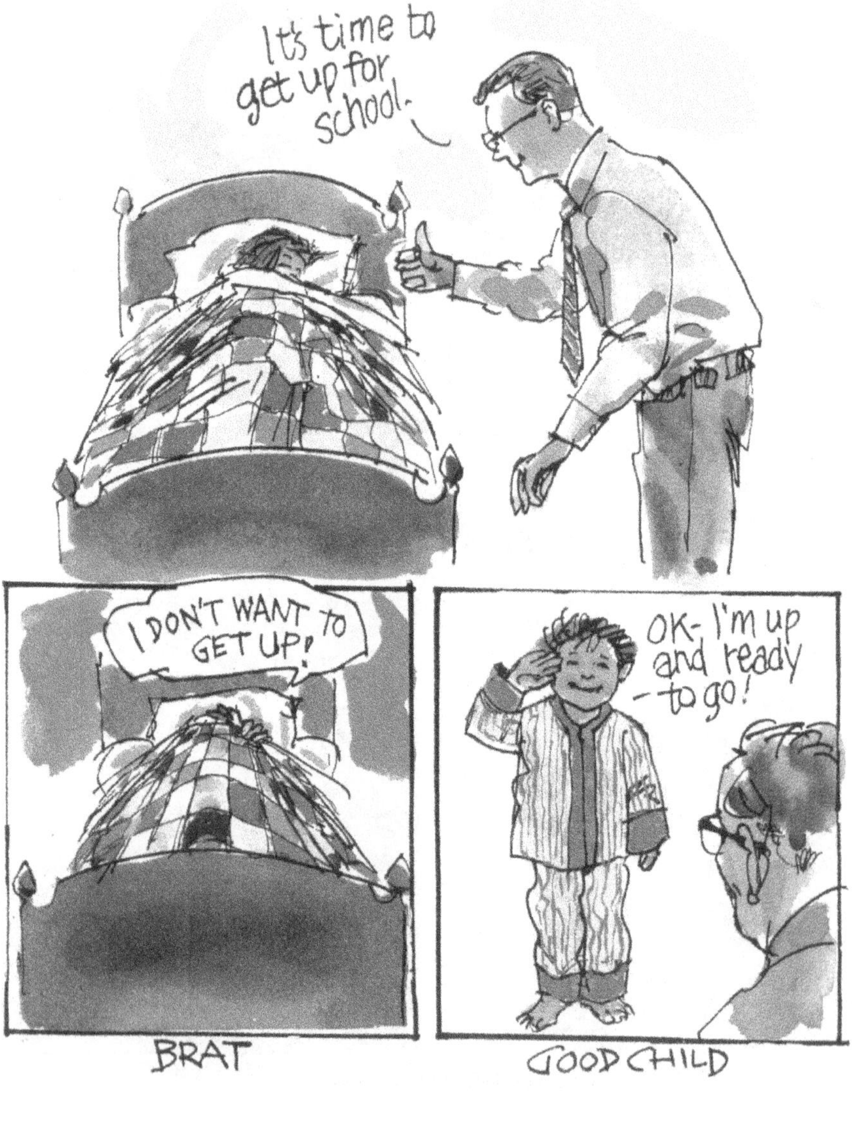
It's time to get up for school.
I DON'T WANT TO GET UP!
OK- I'm up and ready to go!
BRAT
GOOD CHILD

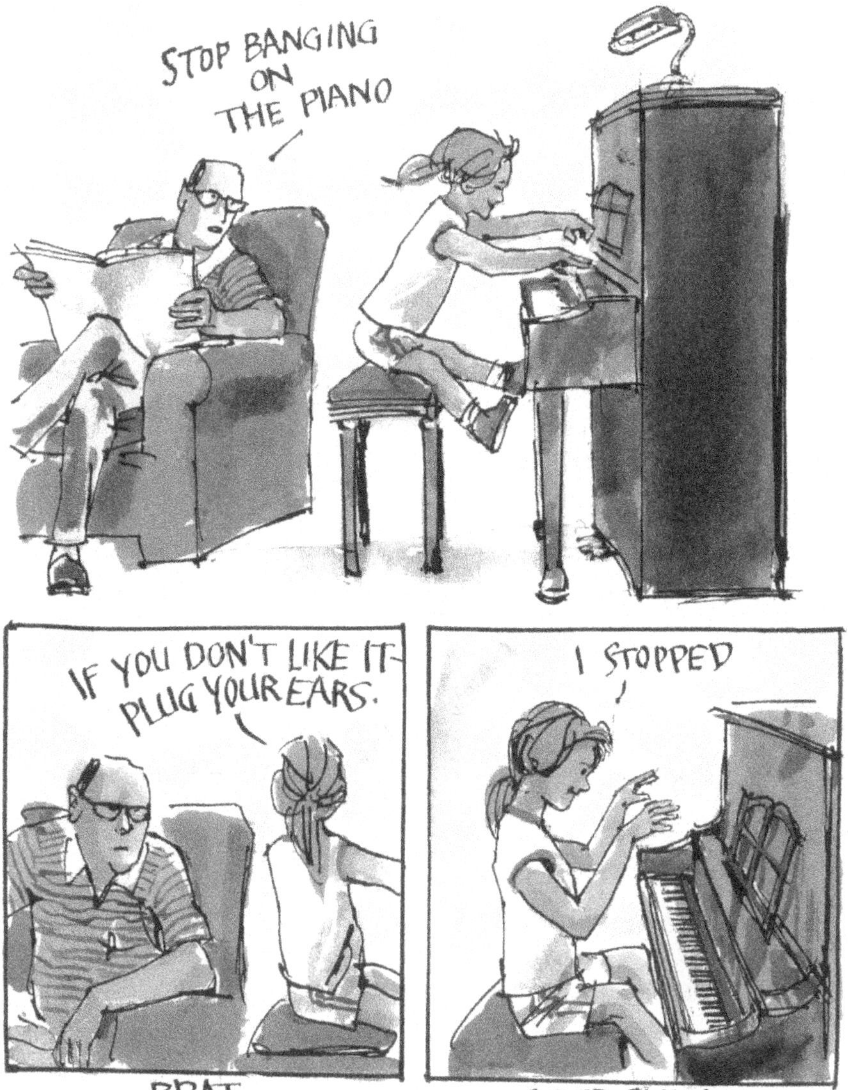
STOP BANGING ON THE PIANO
IF YOU DON'T LIKE IT- PLUG YOUR EARS.
I STOPPED

BRAT

GOOD CHILD

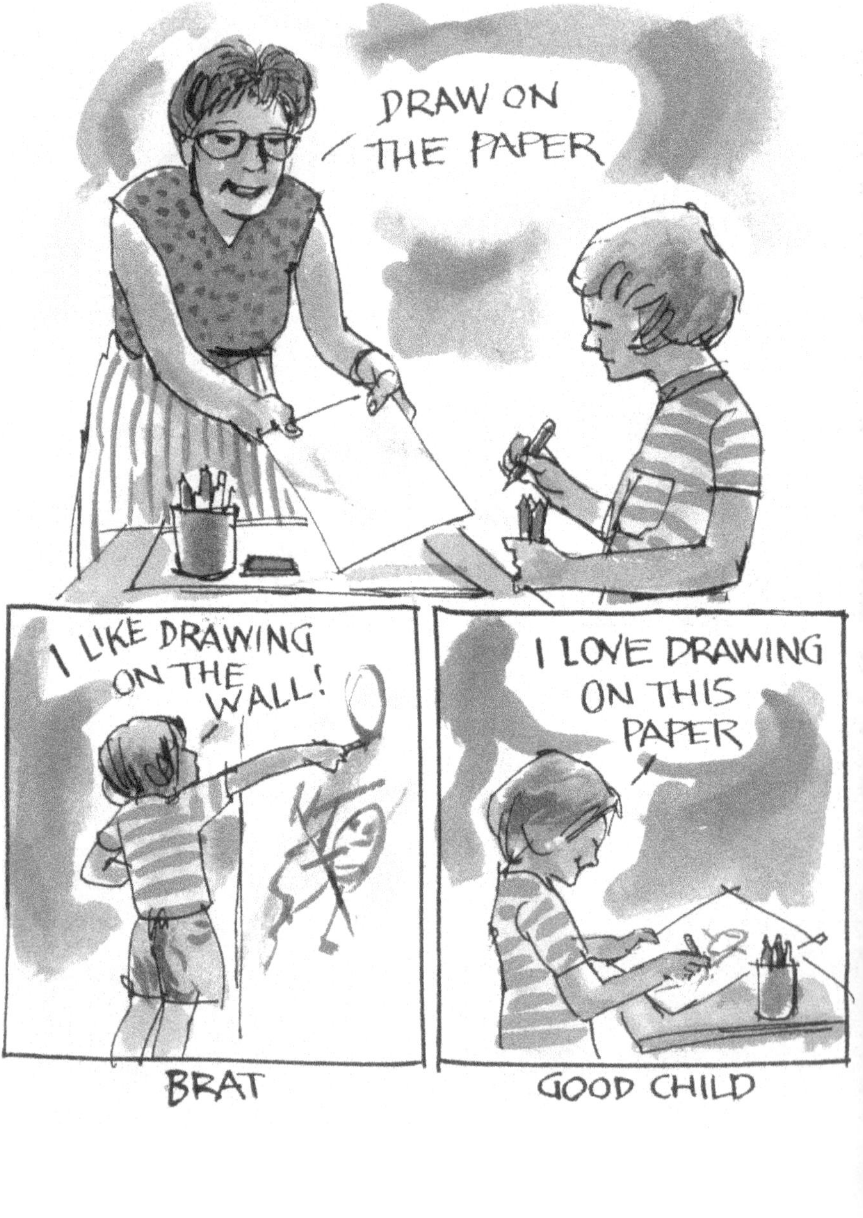
DRAW ON THE PAPER
I LIKE DRAWING ON THE WALL!
I LOVE DRAWING ON THIS PAPER
BRAT
GOOD CHILD

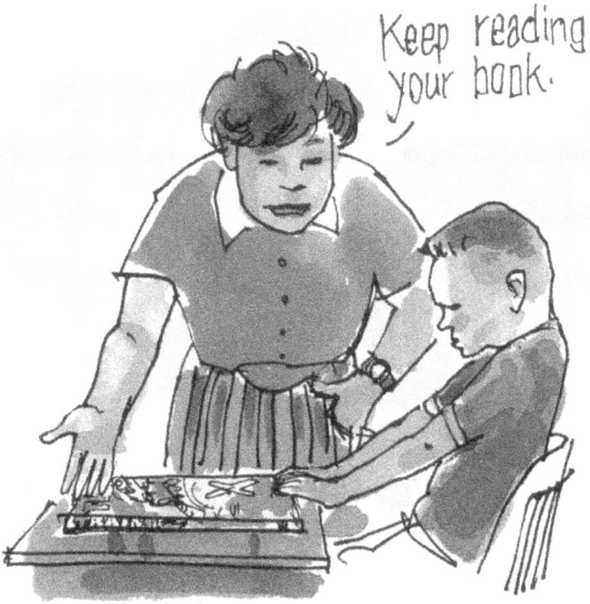
Keep reading your book.

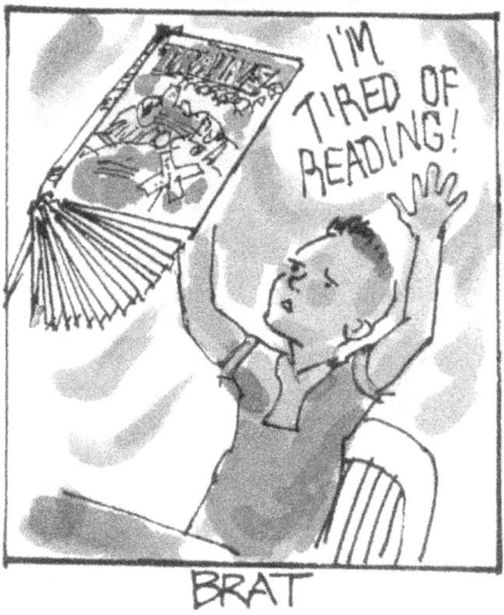
I'M TIRED OF READING!

BRAT

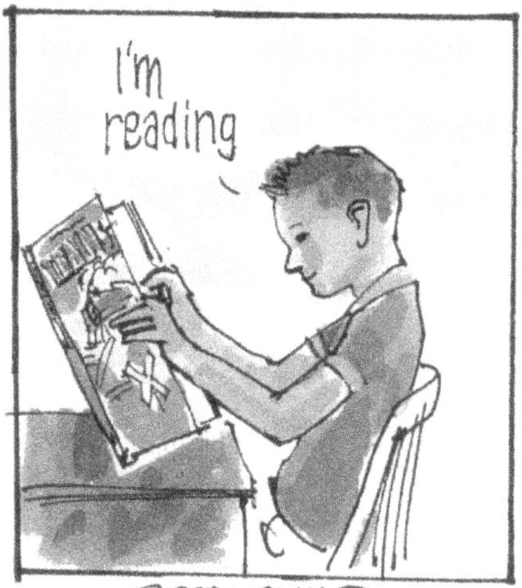
I'm reading

GOOD CHILD

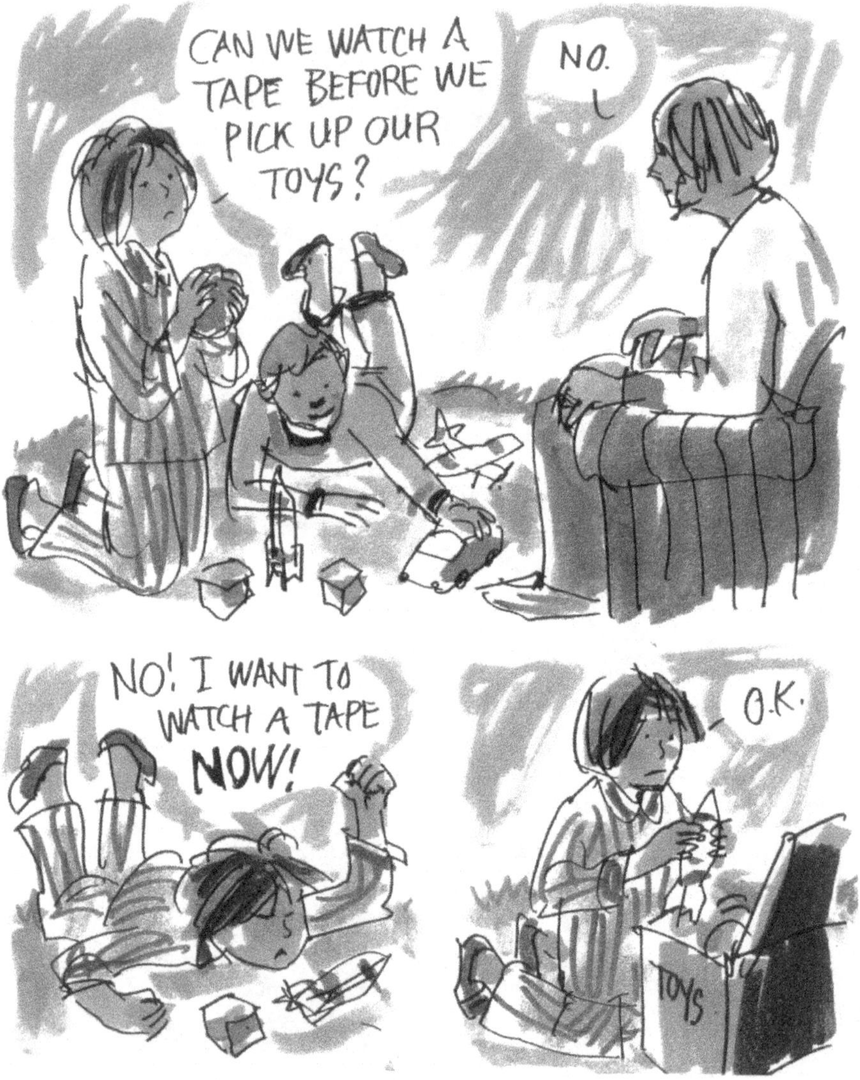
CAN WE WATCH A TAPE BEFORE WE PICK UP OUR TOYS?
NO.
NO! I WANT TO WATCH A TAPE NOW!
O.K.
TOYS

BRAT

GOOD CHILD

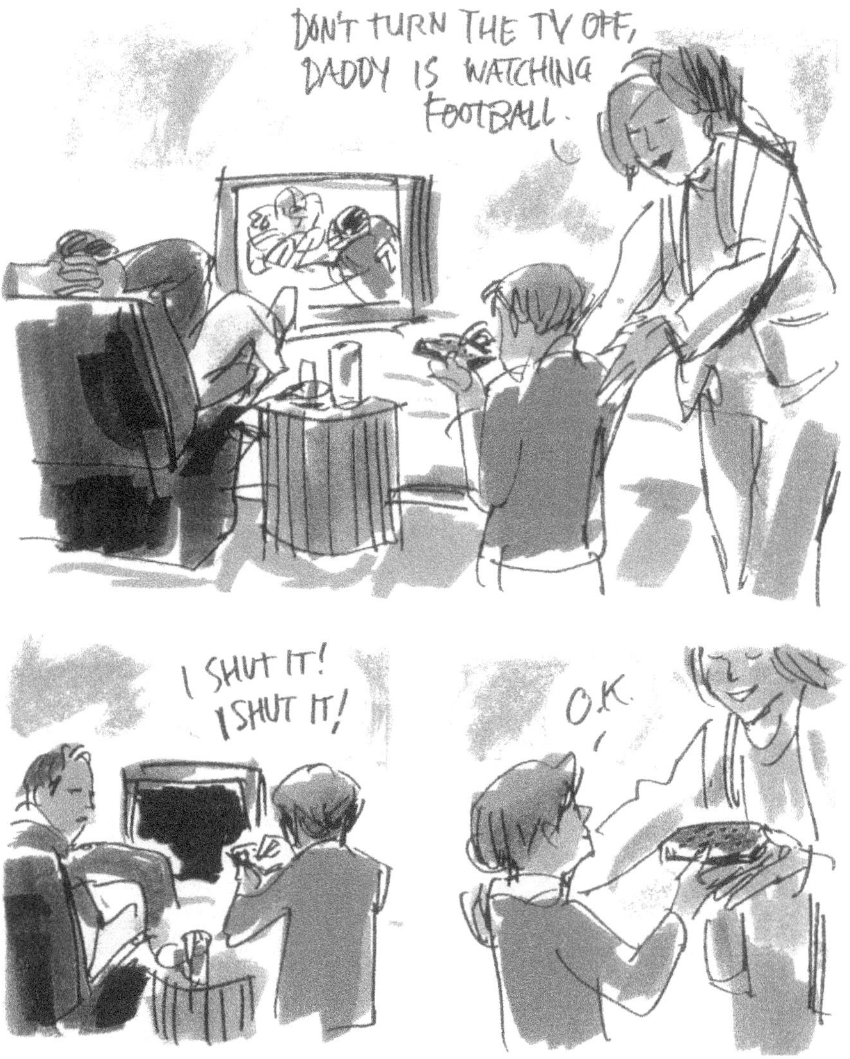

BRAT

GOOD CHILD

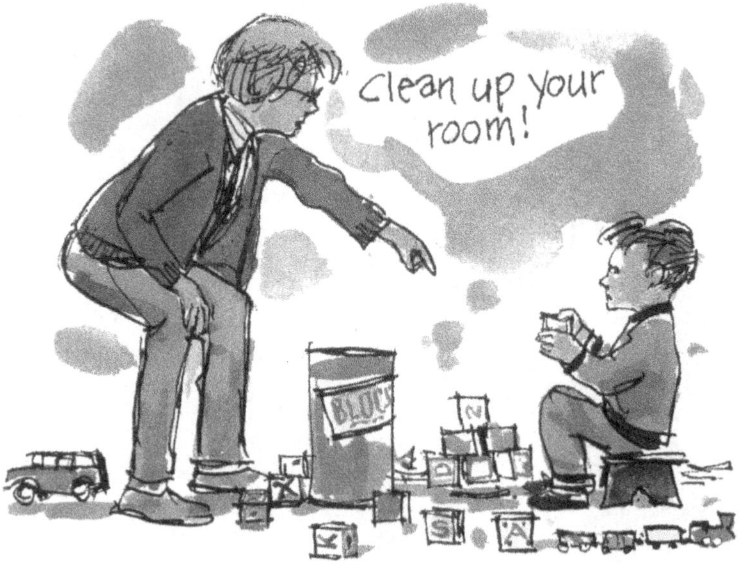

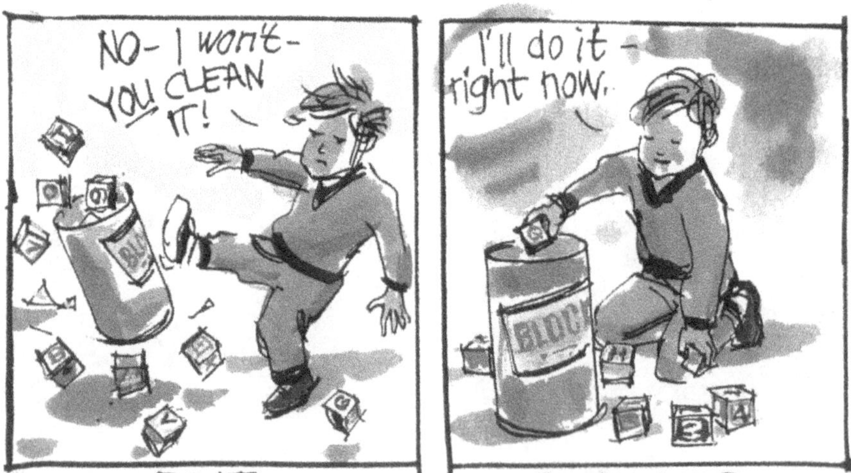

BRAT GOOD CHILD

IV

Communication

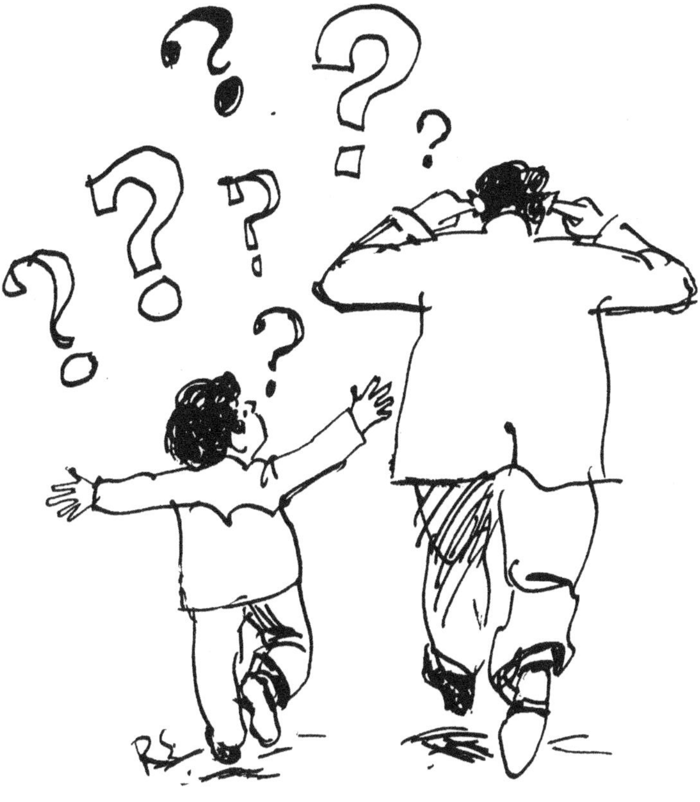

Why? Why? Why? Why?

Communication

Some people make others feel good with just about every communication. The over-gratified will play the "game" of being sweet and soft spoken, pretending to show interest in other people's conversations, becoming popular with everyone except the spouse who is deprived of the luxury of feeling good.
Some people make others feel bad with almost every communication. It's most often intentional, selfish and manipulative.

A comment can have different meanings depending on the pitch, intensity, intonation and volume of the person's voice, as well as the speed of his words. People often experience contradictory feelings about every subject. If one takes a strong position supporting one feeling, it is not unlikely that the listener will take the opposite position. If the answer to the question "Am I upsetting you?" is "No" the unconscious urge may be to try a little harder to upset the person. A person who suffers from a reaction – formation (persistently worrying about someone) casts suspicion that the opposite feeling is hidden from consciousness.

Correctly anticipating the listener's reaction to one's words before the words are uttered shows good judgment. If, on the other hand, the reaction is unexpected, such as a verbal explosion or total silence, the talker's judgment was incorrect. It's best to review the situation and the next time reconsider the approach.

When a person repeatedly complains to someone that he feels mistreated by him, the one being accused must examine what he, in fact, is doing, and regardless of possibly feeling guiltless, there is something he is doing to upset the complainer. To label the one feeling injured as "too sensitive", "imagining it" or "paranoid" is negligent. If something said is perceived by the listener as an attack, regardless of whether it was intended as an attack, it nevertheless <u>was</u> an attack.

The gossiper learns who will listen, and during a seemingly harmless conversation, will include a few comments about another's personal problems, making the sordid details appear a necessary part of the story. Rumors often have a route by which they travel. "It's none of my business" is a set of brakes not often applied by the one who does not wish to listen to gossip. Not stopping the gossiper provides the listener with intimate details about another, which if true, he may have rather not known, and which he can never forget nor verify.

Tears are an expression of anger. A person afraid to verbally express his anger may resort to tears. (In time of sorrow, tears replace the words "I have been abandoned!") When hostile comments evoke tears, it is unlikely that anyone will further "attack" the one who is crying.

Suppressed rage turned inward, not having an outlet, may cause depression. Rage does not evaporate. A person must recognize the existence of rage within himself, then verbalize it in small measures, and finally transform it into creative projects. Rather than change himself, the chronic complainer tries to change everyone and everything around him.

Screaming, yelling and punching as a therapeutic outlet is ineffective, for a person's anger "department" is never empty. Telling someone to freely express his anger is destructive, for no matter how many angry words are unleashed, there will always be more pent-up anger.

The more you explain the less they understand! Many details provide the listener with reasons to disagree, argue, or simply misunderstand. It is tiresome to listen to "endless" words. When a problem is brought up again and again, and the arguments go in "circles", chances are one of the participants is emotionally unstable.

Persuasion is a form of torture for both the persuader and the one being persuaded. It is hard work to try to persuade a skeptic, while resisting an onslaught of unsolicited, persuasive arguments is exhausting. Regardless of who wins, the relationship is strained.

At the other extreme, the very quiet person, not speaking up on any issues, often hoards a volcano of rage for a periodic release at home. Appearing complacent to the outside world, he counts on his family not to betray his dual personality.

Silence can be used as a hostile tool. Deprived of "clearing the air", unable to communicate with one who expresses rage with silence, there is no alternative but to eventually become silent oneself, leaving the misunderstanding unresolved. The unreturned phone call, the unanswered letter, snubbing someone, all are acting-out hostile feelings. A pause of silence before responding to a request, although seemingly innocent, may be experienced as a hostile manipulative moment, leaving the one making the request feel stranded. Silence is a powerful tool which is mostly used by the unanalyzed person to communicate rejection.

In a marriage where one partner uses silence as a means of carrying on a quarrel – where children are used to transmit messages: "Tell your father to ..." – the parent imparts greater hostility toward the children than toward the spouse. Children who are forced to participate in their parents' quarrels are drawn into their parents' private relationship, which is destructive all around.

The person who answers every call has both self-esteem and the ability to politely end undesirable conversations. On the other hand, the person who slams down the phone or who storms out of the room in anger communicates that he is capable of making a momentary decision into a permanent alienation. He is not rewarded by calling him back nor inviting him back. People have words. Animals use their teeth, claws, horns and sounds! A person ending a relationship with a fax announcing: "I want nothing more to do with you", or "I want you out of my life" signals having serious problems. A fax marked "confidential", can nevertheless be read by anyone at the receiving end. Talking about problems, injustices, resentments and hurts and not cutting off all contact is the mature and healthy way to react.

Anger has channels by which it travels without harming its owner or its recipient, whereas expressed in "dirty" looks, silence, screaming, or staying away accomplishes nothing. Repeating angry words in a crescendo of sounds is destructive to everyone. Saying once to the one causing the anger "I am angry at you", is "medicine" which relieves the reactive depression (a depression caused by a reaction to an ongoing situation).

Lengthy phone greetings are cumbersome: "Hello. You have reached the Smiths: Michael, Ellen, Jeremy, Rebecca and Betty. None of us are here right now, but if you leave us a message of any length, we will be sure to call you back as soon as possible. Please leave your number and when it is best to reach you. Thank you very much for calling and have a great day. Good-bye."
In contrast: "You have reached the Smiths. Please leave a message", is respectful of the caller's time.
Having a child record the greeting, leaves the caller in an awkward place when recording a message – as though he is talking to the child.
When recording a lengthy message and at the end quickly leaving one's phone number, the listener may have to replay the entire message several times in order to hear the phone number, an unpleasant exercise.

People take the risk of recording messages which, in certain circumstances, could be legally harmful. Voice mail gives the owner the luxury of knowing what the message is about, while the one leaving the message takes a risk. Some attorneys provide voice mail while advising their own clients not to record themselves on anyone else's voice mail.
When put on hold on the telephone and music is played, the listener has two choices: to listen or to disconnect.
When flipping through dozens of radio stations, it is rare to hear Mozart or other classical music.
Stores and restaurants that play music over loud speakers make the shopper a "captive audience" where, if he dislikes the music, he has two choices, to suffer or to depart.

Some questions solicit the usual polite response, such as when a person asks: "How are you?" "Fine, thank you" is the customary response. Anything other than that or "and how are you?" is out of step in our society. If "lonely", "neglected" or "sick" are substituted for the customary "fine thank you" they fall on deaf ears, for by then the inquirer has walked ten paces in the opposite direction. (To be anything but "fine, thank you" is the quickest way to be avoided.)

Many sentences could be transformed into questions, if the intonation were so placed, thus engaging another in the conversation.

"You know what I mean?" could be responded to with "What do you mean?" (How would anyone know with certainty what another person means?)

Taken literally, a response to the frequently inserted "you know" between sentences, could be "Why are you telling me, if I know?"

The response to the frequent space filler, "I don't know," could be "then why do you keep talking about it if you don't know?"

The person who uses the expression "The truth is" or "To be honest" should be asked: "Was the rest a lie?"

When one says in passing: "I'm not an attorney", or "I'm not a doctor", the listener could respond: "I know. I'm not stupid".

Saying "no problem" when confronted by a big problem is essentially a socially accepted "nice-nice", but often a lie.

The person who says: "Trust me" is presumptuous.

When being served food at a restaurant and told "enjoy", it could be experienced as instructive.

A child only spoken to with loving words, will, when grown up, be unaccustomed to hearing negative comments, and thus may become a compulsive talker, filling spaces between his sentences with "You know", in order to keep the listener from having the opportunity to jump in and possibly saying something hurtful.

Before taking a tough, uncompromising position, a person has to be realistic about what rung on the ladder he is. If a person misjudges his position, he may be setting himself for a tumble. While the fool thinks it over, the wise man thinks it over, too! The person, who postpones an impending agreement in the hope of winning an advantage, will discover that the wise man may use the time to reconsider his own position, which may leave the fool begging to reinstate the former agreement, but to no avail. A man asked a woman he was dating to marry him. She said "no", but a few weeks later she reconsidered. He then turned her down, stating that if she had really wanted to be with him, she would have said "yes" when he asked for her hand in marriage. People who change their minds abruptly without warning could get "run over" like a squirrel who suddenly changes direction without notice. A person whose feelings fluctuate rapidly back and forth, like a strobe light, is emotionally unstable.

Biting one's fingernails symbolically prevents one from scratching the "enemy". In the same way, letting one's teeth rot prevents temptation to "bite" the enemy. Both are symbolic attempts at controlling one's aggression.

Some creative endeavors are forms of communication which are minimized by questions. Forcing the artist to delve into his storeroom of unconscious ideas can disrupt his free expression. An artist questioned about his work may find that in analyzing each line it dilutes his inspiration. Art is a form of communication where the viewer comes up with interpretations. However, interpreting a child's art or asking the child to tell what he drew, are both intrusive. "I like your colors", "You will be an artist", "This looks like your house," are all intrusive comments. If the child volunteers comments about what he drew, one listens in silence. It is best to give the child paper, paints and space to work, whereas telling the child what to draw or taking his pencil and drawing on his work is destructive. Paint-by-number and coloring books are, at best, uncreative and confining. Choosing the best picture among children's drawings is subjective.

Euphemisms as Communication

"I feel sick" is a clear statement. "I feel sick as a dog" lends itself to subjective interpretation depending on the listener's experience.

If words are taken literally, the image conjured by "it's raining cats and dogs" is both unsightly and untruthful.

Euphemisms arouse emotions and images with the use of a few words.

Examples of Euphemisms

The Arts

That painting really isn't my cup of tea. Try as I might to sink my teeth into it, it's a crying shame I can't wax eloquent truth to tell if it's a bitter pill to swallow, a real harebrained low blow which fell between the cracks, if you can see the light and come to your senses. The artist's resting on his laurels trying to show his mettle in a real leap of faith. He's tilting at windmills, if you want to check my crib notes; I've got him pegged. I don't give a fig if this lets the air out of his sails. I'm not going to walk on eggshells or whitewash the issue; I've got an eye for the goods and know a diamond in the rough when push comes to shove. I wouldn't give a king's ransom for this brick he threw up which I'm not going to handle with kid gloves. Call it nitpicking, call it hot-dogging; he's got to learn from the school of hard knocks that I wasn't born yesterday and take it to heart that it'll all come out in the wash, that his piece is really a house of cards that he'd better learn to keep time. This isn't a tongue lashing; beauty is in the eye of the beholder, I know how to mind my P's and Q's; time to cut bait and put one foot in front of the other and say to himself "no guts, no glory"; Right now it doesn't fly and he's gotta follow advice and be a chip off the old block of the old school.

Crime

I almost cashed in my chips when the heat really let it fly and a .22 almost popped me in the noodle. I got out of there by a whisker but I was cool as a cucumber and hung in there even though I was left holding the bag. I was quaking in my boot and out on a limb, to make a mountain out of a molehill. I only did it to try to make ends meet, but it got out of hand and I found myself in quite a pickle, even though I split hairs and was letter perfect when I stepped into the limelight and staked my claim. I had my eyes peeled though I felt hot under the collar and though my goose was cooked when that gave me lip. I got it all squared away though; I went from the spot on top of the world, and thought of all of them with cold feet who ratted on this sting operation. I'll never warm up to them, the drips! Wake up and smell the coffee! Get a grip! You gotta roll with the punches and stop this hemming and hawing – it's as easy as pie.

Don't give me a song and dance when you don't have two nickels to rub together! I'm between a rock and a hard place too, you know. Just get your ducks lined up in a row and you won't be like a deer caught in the headlights sticking it's neck out for a tonguelashing. Look at me, riding high! I'm all fired up and got my pie in the sky! Like taking candy from a baby!

The Gourmet

My cup runneth over. ... I'm about to step up to the plate and chow down in this there dining car with this beef that I don't have a beef with ... Dollars to doughnut that this ain't no red herring even if you don't give a fig whether I stiff the waiter or not. I'm not hot-dogging, let me tell you, I'm chopping at the bit to wolf down these ears of corn and you know I drink like a fish. Frankly I enjoy being waited on hand and foot and give a roast as good as I get; don't egg me on. Believe me, I'm not biting the hand that feeds me or looking a gift horse in the mouth, You scratch my back and I'll scratch yours, and this is my just reward. This place is quite a watering hole, a whole other kettle of fish; no sour grapes on my part. Anyhow, my job is cut out for me because I've got a lot on my plate. They said if you can't stand the heat get out of the kitchen, so here I am licking my chops and plum crazy over this table set for me. Forgive me for being so schmaltzy but I know who my meal ticket is so here's to you and me; two peas in a pod.

Man, I'm jerkin' around, barkin' up the wrong tree. I'm seein' stars 'cuz I'm brown-nosing up this ball breaker like the bees to honey, She's uh, she's uh, she's nothin' but jail bait an' I'm sittin' here chasin' rainbows. I better cut this out before I burst my bubble. Come here, no, maybe you shouldn't 'cuz I'm gonna' rain on your parade. It's all nothing but a lemon. I'm gonna lay all my cards on the table. Damn, these dog days of summer. I tell you she's stacked. I don't know how I'm gonna grab the bull by the horns. When push come to shove, I'm a sucker. My days are numbered; I'm waitin' for the other shoe to drop. Shoo, I'm workin' like a dog. I'm in a pickle. Feelin' blue. I've got to swallow my pride, iron out the differences and cash in my chips. Don't fence me in. I'm about to curb my loins and turn the table on someone. 'Cuz the shit has hit the fan and I ain't gettin' the lion's share. I'll tell you what. I am gettin' the lion's share of the kiss of death 'cuz this stuff is like pullin' teeth and I'm sick of twistin' his arm. I've bit off more than I can chew. I'm just scrapin' bottom right now. I'll tell you what. My cup ain't exactly runneth over. I smell a rat. I smell a rat. I ain't about to let sleepin' dogs lie. I'm tired of this horsin' around. I've been jumpin' through hoops and I ain't no more cold as a cucumber. This ain't no bed of roses. I'm about to turn over a new leaf in one fail swoop. I'd rather do that than kick the bucket. It's time for me to cut and run and paper over the differences. I'm speakin' with a forked tongue. No more nickel and dimein' someone. No more goin' out on a limb. I'm gonna' quit stallin' and put that in my pipe and smoke it. I'm not gonna make a mountain out of a molehill no more.

I'm in my cups I've gotta' beefs, 'cuz I'm stuck on someone I've been tiltin at windmills, I'm scrappin' the bottom of the barrel here. Paintin' myself into a corner in spades, shoot, I've gotta wake up and smell the coffee and give somebody the slip. Brush somebody off. She's runnin' me ragged. I'm hang dog. I've got tunnel vision over this. I can't gloss over this. She's houndin' on me. I'm not sittin' on a fence. I, I, I I'm about to strike out. I'm bein' run circles on. I don't rest on my laurels; I ain't three sheets to the wind no more. I, I, don't got it made in the shade, I'm off to the races. I've got a crush on someone. Damn, time I saw the light. I've gotta see the forest for the trees. And punch in and give somebody hell. You know the score? I've gotta come to my senses. I fell between the cracks. I betcha dollars to donuts. I take my hat off to the person 'cuz I've got him pegged. He's drinkin' me under the table and he made it look as easy as pie. Damn, man, he's drivin' me bananas. This a jam session. I'm not gonna beat around the bush. 'Cuz I threw up a brick. I've gotta hand it to him. This guy's a diamond in the rough. This is an open and shut case. I stuck my neck out and I bit the bullet. Right now I'm at loggerheads 'cuz I'm floundering' and I'm at rope's end and I'm fit to be tied. 'Cuz I don't give a fig no more. I can't walk in somebody else's shoes. This guy reinvented the wheel and now I've got to handle him with kid gloves. And I ain't gonna box his ears. I tried to let the air out of his sails. I died with my boots on. I ain't got a ghost of a chance. I ain't no chip off the old block. Now, she says to me "Don't take it to heart" what does she think? I was born yesterday? Stop pullin' my leg. I know I smoke like a chimney. I got myself in hot water. Anyway, what she was tellin' me was music to my ears. Even though she said I'm nuts and that's bologna. She ain't gonna come near me with a ten foot pole. But I don't care about any of that 'cuz birds of a feather gotta stick together. You don't give me a song and dance anymore. It's time to balance the budget.

And, I've been goin' overboard and tryin' to count my chickens before they hatch. And that makes people cop an attitude and instead of that I'm gonna toe the line and stop this clownin' around and drive it home. And blank out, blank out this gettin' myself in a pickle. Time I got quiet as a mouse and got through these dog days of summer. An' pay the piper, I'm gonna sleep on it and keep on truckin', and doin' the old soft shoe and maybe beat a hasty retreat. When push comes to shove it'll all come out in the wash,

(*English accent:*) On a hop, skip and a jump, it's time I spilled my guts. For the life of me this thing's gotten out of hand and all things aren't being equal. It's not on a back burner anymore. We're two ships in the night and this thing's giving me a pain in the neck 'cuz I'm over a barrel this is not something that is pretty as a picture. I'm fighting the elements and I'm trying to come up with a keynote address and the cat's got my tongue, really. And even though I've been going at it tooth and nail and I'm trying to mind my P's and Q's, but to be honest I've been talking a mile a minute, and I've got a little bit of sour grapes here trying to shoot the breeze. Instead this is a whole other kettle of fish. No longer am I sharp as a whip. I've been trying to sink my teeth into it and to be quite honest, I don't have two nickels to rub together, and I really don't want to look a gift horse in the mouth.

My son, I ain't fired with enthusiasm, 'cuz I got my job cut out for me, you know, I ain't got no information at my fingertips. By trying to walk in-between the raindrops and what do you do? You come over here an' knock my teeth in. I'm at the end of my rope an' I'm startin' to clam up man, you know? Come here. Come here I want to steal a minute 'cuz I'm crazy about you man. You know the strings attached, you know? Don't throw the baby out with the bath water. NO. You know this ain't no needle in a haystack. Ya got to stick with your guns man and get off my back, man. You got to put one foot in front of the other and don't give me the time of day. 'Cuz you know you can't walk in somebody else's shoes. And beggars can't be choosers. An' I'm all fired up. Don't give' me the evil eye, no.

I got to toe the line? An' you think I was born yesterday? No. I'm not about to get green, take it to heart or get bent out of shape. I've been to the school of hard knocks. I know how to dish out the dirt and uh, I got my sea legs now, see, I laid down the law and done fed 'em a line. Then I beat a hasty retreat and keep on truckin' to try an' pan somethin' to pay the piper. And sleep on it. I got myself in a pickle but it fits like a glove and these are the dog days of summer. Even though I'm still skatin' on thin ice and about to jump out of my skin but it'll all come out in the wash.

This is my bread and butter then the chickens are gonna come home to roost an' I'll be cool as a cucumber. On the dime. No dead beat dad 'cuz the writin's on the wall. Then I can dish it out in a bedside manner and can shoot the breeze.

Ok here we go. This should be up your alley. I'm gonna weave a story even though I feel like I'm runnin' on empty. So, don't put the brakes on 'cuz all things being equal, I don't want you to crawl into a hole. This ain't no freebie so you gotta jump through hoops. For me it's a sweatshop 'cuz I get carried away 'cuz, you know, I'm the breadwinner. Sometimes it's a bitter pill to swallow. Don't cop an attitude. OK? Now this is a groundbreaking event and I don't want you to get cagey or make this a bone of contention. No more penny pinching now. OK a little bit of tongue and cheek. You better run for cover 'cuz I'm about to bum your bridges. Come on, come on and touch base with me and put your best foot forward. 'Cuz you think it's in the bag. You think, I want you to give me your best shot. Teacher's pet stuff. I'm ridin' my high horse and see my teeth are as white as pearls and I'm about to dive into my chicken soup in hindsight. I fly off the handle. So you better give me some hush money before I start blowin' your horn and I'm gonna burst with pride. So I'm gonna leave you in the dust 'cuz the sky's the limit and I'm about to straiten up and fly right. You get between the covers this ain't no dead-end. I ain't runnin' on empty. And you can take that with you. Beauty is only skin deep miss crybaby. You better hold your tongue and don't look that gift horse in the mouth. Just cut your losses 'cuz we're strange bedfellows and you bit off more than you could chew. Don't get me wrong, I'm not off the top of my head. Nor did I get up on the wrong side of the bed. You better sink your teeth into it. You know from soup to nuts I'm sharp as a tack. I ain't moonstruck, even though I know I'm the apple of her eye, I'm facin' the music even though it's between a rock and a hard place. This is my keynote address. I'm busy as a bee and snug as a bug in a rug. I'm about to talk a blue streak. And don't tell me this is a house of cards, miss stuffed shirt. I'm not piggin' out. I'm just going at it tooth and nail and getting' the dirt on 'em.

It's time to shoot the breeze. I'm about to speak my mind and don't call me no paper tiger nor devil's advocate just 'cuz I went out and painted the town red. 'Cuz I thought it was a sound investment. You hear me talking a mile a minute you ain't gonna hear nothing about no sour grapes 'cuz I got the lions share, you won't find me green with envy even though I'm shootin' the breeze and givin' you a tongue lashing. Well let me hold on. I better make it slow as molasses 'cuz I've been straight as an arrow and dead pan so don't hold your breath.

Sit a spell. It's time to get carried away. You are missing your mark and you better hang in there big cheese. You're gonna be up a creek in quite a dish. Don't jump the gun, it's time to kick his ass. Steal yourself, and play hookey 'cuz you're on the horn of a dilemma. If you cross paths and turn into a stock character, when push comes to shove. It's cut check time and time to file memo. Don't be easily swayed. Better dot your i's and cross your t's. Get over the hump and stop flogging a dead horse. I'm not talking below me I'm not jerking around. I'm not being crabby. It's time to get back to the drawing board and take a load off. Get on the right track and stop being a pain in the neck. If you need an extra pair of hands. Give me a break. I'm in the doghouse. I'm about to hit sec? I'm on the beam when push comes to shove. I've been pouring over this Mr. Letter Perfect. I'm not going to paper over the differences. I'm not speaking with a forked tongue. I ain't kickin' a fuss. It's time to turn the tables on someone.

Give me hell. Make it snappy. On the double. Stop it. I'm gonna run out of steam. It's as plain as the nose on your face. I'm flexing my muscles. It's not a running gag anymore. It's cast in stone, dammit! Nothing to sneeze at. So, get your shit together!

Before you get a backlash and get out of the heat, this ain't no barrel of fun for me. I'm out in left field. I ain't bullish on this no, no sir this is my bread and butter and I'm just gonna stake my claim. Because of this, I'm not having a whale of a time. I'm about to give you a knuckle sandwich. I'm gonna bolt and cable someone. I've got to kick this habit. I got cold feet. And you think this is a fountain of youth? No, I ain't stilted and I've been pushing the envelope so don't call me an ambulance chaser. I'm died in the wool, been eaten alive. Keep going. Scratch the surface. Play the field. Just out of the blue you say I'm out of line. Even though we're just chewing the fat. You told me a word to the wise about holy matrimony and I started to clam up, even though I thought I was on a roll. I was sproutin' up and you wired me and my feet turned into clay. I saw it was a bait and switch and I started getting cold turkey and saw this ain't my cup of tea. I can't get a handle on it even though I was wax and eloquent. I was about to sweep it under the rug. Then decided to get a Gypsy cab and was thrown for a loop.

V

Truth

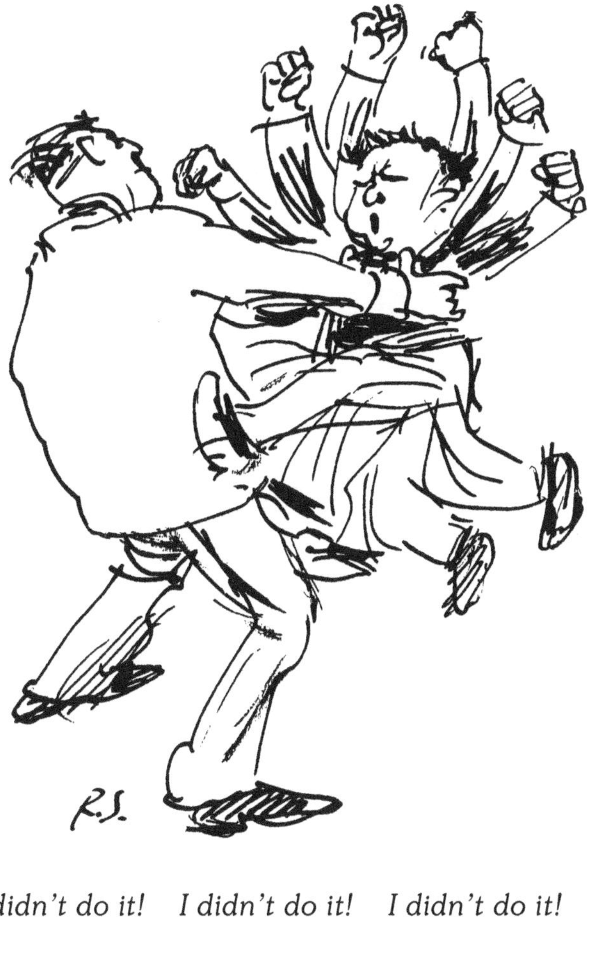

I didn't do it! I didn't do it! I didn't do it!

Truth

A liar who begins to believe his own lies will act incensed when suspected of being a liar. A person who lies once is no longer trustworthy. White lies are still lies. There is only one truth, and getting in trouble for telling the truth is a compliment because of the promise of learning to walk the straight and narrow.
Telling a lie often weaves a stream of lies, one covering another. As one's memory fades, trust goes out the window. Thievery in the human race is monumental. Partners are stolen, ideas are stolen and possessions are stolen. Animals steal the eggs of other species. Carnivorous animals and people kill and eat their prey.

The ability of man and woman to create a baby is beyond comprehension. Can a pregnant mother consciously direct the forming of the baby's organs, limbs etc.? Once born, does the baby's conscious mind direct the digesting of food and how to turn some of it into blood, some of it into urine and some of it gets defecated? Who tells the body what and how to do it? When at sixteen weeks of pregnancy an amnio reveals the sex of the embryo and the parents elect to wait and be surprised to find out the truth at the moment of birth, they don't fully accept the embryo for who he/she is until birth. The surprise could be equally exciting at sixteen weeks.

If people steal, if they lie, they should be brought to justice. However, looking at the complete picture, the fault lies with their parents, or whoever brought them up to feel entitled, and if they don't get something, they steal. If they get away with telling a lie, they tell lies. The message they received as they grew up was: "Do whatever will make you happy. If it makes you happy to steal, steal". Children who were brought up to feel entitled, where honesty is discarded, will, as adults, do all kinds of terrible things, which could get them in trouble with the law. Their parents, while trying to make them happy, unintentionally ruined their lives.

The overindulged feels entitled, helping himself to whatever he wants, crossing boundaries of honesty, while thinking that everyone around is too stupid to notice that he is, in fact, a thief, a liar and an actor. When an honest person is careless about his possessions, it tempts the overindulged dishonest person to steal. Sensing his victim has become aware of the theft, the thief, in order not to be discovered and having no conscience, adds insult to injury and accuses his victim of being "paranoid". The thief steals both material possessions and his victim's good reputation. Anyone can say anything derogatory about anyone and, regardless if it is only partially true or not true at all, some of it "sticks". Since one's reputation travels with one forever, a person can be harmed by untruths spread about him. The guilty person deserving of the academy award, once accused of thievery, will not only act guiltless but also incensed, cutting off all contact with the one he stole from! When an innocent person is accused of thievery, he will deny the accusation and not make an issue of it.

Should children be taught that there are acceptable lies such as Santa Claus coming down the chimney, the stork bringing the baby, the tooth fairy leaving money under the pillow, and the Easter Bunny laying eggs?
When playing a game with one's child, parents who manipulate the game so the child wins, teach the child dishonesty along with entitlement. Lying to a child, such as agreeing to come home at a certain time and then arriving much later, or promising to stay home and then leaving after the child falls asleep, sets a poor example. A parent who is an unfaithful promiscuous spouse, although keeping it all secretive, will find that his children's unconscious picks up the perverted behavior, which they may imitate.

Teaching children that they can get whatever they want, sends them on a lifetime entitlement voyage. They lie, they steal, they are fakes. They look very sweet and behave in a way that people think they are wonderful. They actually tell themselves something to feel okay about stealing, about lying and all the deceptions. Perhaps what they say to themselves is: "Mommy and Daddy told me I should be happy and that I deserve everything because I'm so wonderful. I am merely obeying their advice."

A liar has no conscience that monitors him. To protect himself he will deceive others and resort to damaging the reputation of another, while protective of his parents whom he counts on to indulge him to the last day of his life. Unless a person has a vigilant and punitive super-ego – a conscience that monitors him – anything goes!

Dishonesty takes many forms, including lying, stealing, deceiving, pretending and acting. For example, if the boss signals: "I'm not here!", and the secretary's response to a caller who asks to speak to the boss is: "He is away from his desk," or "He is on a conference call" after that, how can the secretary and boss trust each other? They are partners in deception.

A deceptive insurance representative who answered her secretary's phone received a call from a person asking to speak to her! Not informing the caller that she, in fact, was that person, she responded: "I can give you her voice mail", and did! Directing a caller to voice mail, a substitute for speaking to a person, could be interpreted as an avoidance, unless the call is returned.

The overindulged child grows up knowing how to sniff out a naive host who will be fooled and emotionally coerced into becoming obligated to help, rescue and support the manipulative parasite. It's an on-going tragic saga for the host who cannot emotionally, physically or financially disconnect from, or abandon the parasite who uses charm and deception to stay leached onto the host, sucking up his "last" penny. A victim unable to dislodge himself from the manipulative trap will become a lifelong slave to the manipulator who knows how to "push his buttons".

Giving, as a form of obligating, is emotional bribery. Falling into this predicament, the taker ends up giving much more than he receives. A gift, its timing and the manner in which it is given reveals much more about the giver. On the other hand, the chronic taker, manipulative and opportunistic in nature, feigning modesty, makes the giver feel apologetic for not having given more.

The rich who don't pay their bills on time impart that they think that everyone has money. It is a reckless lack of understanding and concern. When it comes to revealing how much money one earns or has accumulated, most people are secretive, fearing it will be "taken away".

A person instrumental in helping someone achieve success should get credit and financial reward. Too often the successful neglect to share the rewards with the enablers.
A man wrote a book about how a father should interact with his children. Because of anger at the way his own father related to him, he left his father's name out. However, his father gave him life, and ability to write a book about child rearing. He should have thanked his father for not overindulging him, and as a result he was able to use his talents to write a book.

One woman did not want her children to find out that she was several years older than their father, so she lied about her age, and took the deception to extremes. She never told her children that she was a college graduate, so when she went to her college reunions she pretended she was joining her husband on his reunions – since they both attended the same school. It wasn't until many years later, when she died, that the adult children read in the obituary her true age. The father cooperated with the deception, thereby unintentionally teaching their children deception.

A college drama instructor gave the students a perverse and intrusive assignment of secretly jotting down a conversation between unsuspecting strangers, who were unaware of being eavesdropped.

One young boy believed his stepmother was his biological mother, until the stepmother left his father, and the boy became upset. At that point the older siblings calmed him down with the truth they had known all along, informing him that who he thought was his biological mother was, in fact, his stepmother. After that deception – it was difficult for him to trust ever again.

An insightful theory of dreams, elegant in its simplicity, inspired a therapist to write a book. She asked her supervisor if he would join her in co-authoring and substantiating her theory. He listened attentively, and seemed quite interested. "Yes," of course he would help her put together a book. But several months later he changed his mind and then came the phone call. A betrayal so deep that it pierced her like a mortal wound. He had decided to lecture about her dream theories and not give her credit and if she didn't agree, there would be consequences: He would never speak to her again. He asked her to sign a note of agreement which he was about to send to her. She said she would write it herself and send it to him, but was advised by her medical doctor not to. Upon not receiving the note the supervisor told the therapist's son that his mother was a liar for not sending him the release. She then had no proof of his intended plagiarism as she began work on her book. As she was about to publish, his defenses grew. Afraid that she would expose him, he slandered her, trying to discredit her, her character and her ability as a therapist, so that if she were to reveal his intended plagiarism, no one would believe her.

VI
"Whatever Makes You Happy"

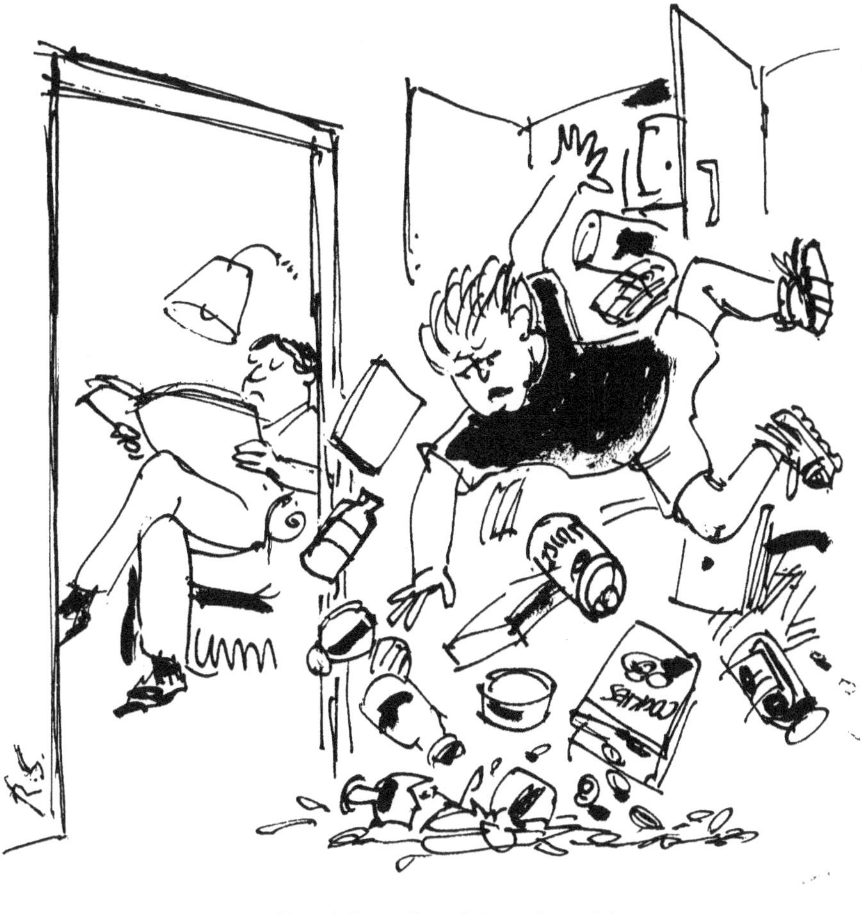

Crash! *Crash!* *Crash!*

“Whatever Makes You Happy”

Parents who tell their children: “All I want for you is to be happy in life” are giving them an impossible assignment, since happiness is elusive and, at best, intermittent. When these children grow up they will flounder from profession to profession looking for the one profession that will make them happy. They will have difficulty settling down with one partner as they search for happiness. It’s an unachievable assignment and, ironically, a life sentence of unhappiness.

People whose preoccupation in life is happiness, too often abuse alcohol, smoke and overeat. They are remise in not understanding that just being alive is fun and that in their pursuit of superficial fun they cut their lives short.
When seeking happiness by overeating, the person no longer savors what’s in his mouth, unless there’s more on his plate to look forward to. The three T’s – texture, temperature and taste – combine into a yearning for a particular food.
Opera singers are often obese – overindulgence has taken over. They give out many sounds through their mouth which are then replaced with food. In a similar way, the person who habitually reads while defecating on the toilet, symbolically replaces the “loss” by “taking in” through his eyes.
In this country each holiday begins with pre-holiday preparation and ends with post-holiday recuperation, where the country is “shut down” for three days or more, where work, school and government come to a halt. It’s all about fun! fun! fun!

Repeatedly told: “Do whatever makes you happy”, once grown, the person tries to figure out: “What do I want to do with my life other than what I’m doing? Do I want a different job? Do I want a different profession? Do I want to re-invent myself?” Hopelessly lost, some missing piece stands in the way of “What do I really want to do that will make me happy, instead of what I am doing?" The person has no clear idea of what new profession to pursue. No clue.

What would break the cycle – which must be done early in the child's life – is the provision of clear parental direction; e.g.: "I want you to become a doctor!" (not: "You'd be a very good doctor!"). The first is a command, the second is over-gratification. The child who grows up obeying the parents' commands copes with life, while the one regularly complemented ends up in the corner with a symbolic pacifier in his mouth, whimpering: "I want mommy!"

Children grow up aimless if parental direction is not provided for them via forthright communication. These children are not obligated to follow their parents' direction, but it nevertheless sets forth a clear plan. By young adulthood, they should have developed the capacity to navigate life's decisions with a greater sense of independence and self-awareness. But the "whatever makes you happy" philosophy does not provide the impetus. Parents who say: "I have no idea what would make my child happy!" point to an ongoing problem passed from generation to generation, namely, that it doesn't make the parent happy to upset his child by telling him what profession to pursue.

Parents who put forth an act of always being happy, bring up children who lack empathy, never having had the opportunity to develop empathy for their parents. If they do not learn it from home first, chances are more remote they will learn it from their peers.

The enjoyment, rather than empathy of another's tragedy is predominately what tabloids thrive on. The overindulged will search for a better job, a better partner, a better analyst, and will come up with endless schemes in pursuit of elusive goals. If he fails in accomplishing his own interests and needs, his prime concern becomes that of keeping someone else from getting ahead. Lifting himself up by pushing someone else down, gives a false and perverse feeling of success. A person able to use his eyes to see around him makes every minute worth living, while the miserably unhappy person may exert energy trying to keep others from succeeding. To improve oneself takes thought, plan, hard work and creativity. To destroy someone else takes bitterness, scheming and deceptiveness.

The overindulged child having been repeatedly told he was special grows up expecting his name in lights. Becoming deceptive and dishonest in order to achieve success and ownership of possessions, he will never give credit to someone who helped him achieve success. If unable to achieve his goal, he will become jealous, while rejoicing when tragedies befall another. Having been told: "All I want you to be is happy in life", he manipulates others while being dishonest, which go hand in hand with crossing many boundaries in pursuit of "happiness".

It's about time our society understood that parents of criminals should stand trial, because from day one, these parents provided their children with psychological pacifiers, never permitting them to feel hunger or pain, causing them to grow up unequipped to deal with frustration, putting them on the road to breaking the law and committing crimes. Parents rarely make the connection between the way they raised their children and how their children turned out.

Parents of a nine year old girl who stabbed to death her eleven year old friend while fighting over a ball, should be put on trial for raising an out of control criminal. A man diagnosed with HIV spat into the eyes and mouth of an officer who was arresting him. If parents of such criminals were held legally responsible for their offspring's crimes, they may reconsider the danger of overindulgence.

An elderly mother sued her adult daughter for borrowing money from her and never returning it, not recognizing that it was her fault for bringing up an irresponsible dishonest daughter.

One woman controlled her parents throughout her life with temper tantrums. If she didn't get her way with crying, screaming and stomping her feet she would threaten to go to the bay and drown herself, causing her parents, afraid she'd hurt herself, to give in every time.

VII
Divorce

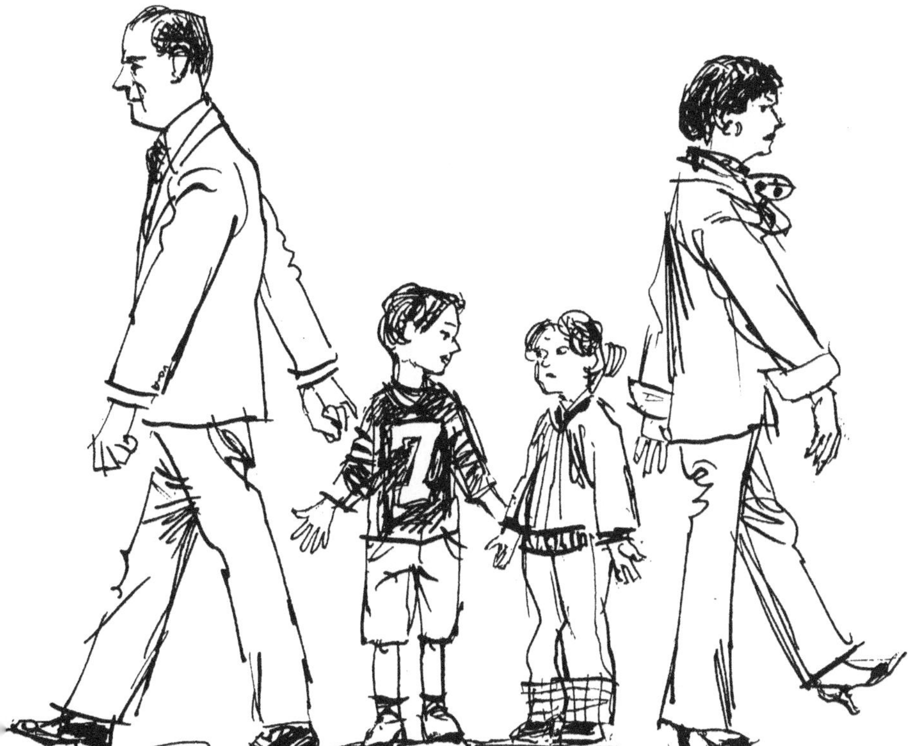

Divorce

Two people with different approaches to money, sex, raising children, religion, one likes it warm, the other likes it cold, one sleeps late, the other rises with the sun, are supposed to live together in harmony.

Before a couple gets married there are always hints and clues of what each partner is going to be like, yet after the couple is married for several months or years each partner often claims: "I had no idea he (or she) was going to be like this". But the fact is, if they think back (a painful process), they will recall that they had clear hints and clues of what the partner would be like. One person deceptively hides flaws, while the other implicitly looks the other way, and vice versa, and in due time, the true nature of the partners inevitably comes to the surface.

It is how they deal with having been deluded in the first place which may eventually send them on the path to divorce. Often disregarding clues of impending serious incompatibility, the young couple nevertheless proceeds into marriage, only to spew surprise and frustration at the unpleasant habits and traits that show up later. All excuses do not cover up the fact that a person was aware, on some level, of what the partner would be like.

When a person decides to file for divorce, too often the one being divorced knows how to manipulate the partner, claiming that it's a mistake, causing the divorce to be postponed, reconsidered or dragged on and on.

In a divorce where one partner deserves the academy award for pretending, the decent partner, not infrequently, gets blamed for the divorce. A deceptive person has two faces: one for the outside world and one for the spouse, who suffers from living with a two-faced fraudulent, soft-spoken fake. In divorces where the fake partner comes off sweet, and the decent partner does not resort to revealing the fake partner's duplicitous nature, the result is that the outside world frequently falls for the act, and instead of blaming the fake, will blame the decent genuine partner for the divorce. A mediocre person often slams the door on the face of the talented. As a result, mediocrity reigns.

Spreading gossip and untruths about the partner to justify the filing for divorce, is a damaging intrusion. The gossiper unwittingly reveals more about himself than about the one he is maligning. He reveals that his problems are so insurmountable that he must distract himself by talking about someone else's problems and that his rage is so overbearing that he must release bits of it at the expense of hurting someone else's reputation.

An older woman had a stroke and moved in with her daughter. A hired nurse reported that the daughter's husband was making sexual advances toward her. The nurse was fired, but the husband continued his philandering with a switch-board operator in his office which finally ended the marriage. Forever after, her neighbors shunned her and didn't greet her, treating her like a criminal for divorcing her husband. The best defense is an offense. However, to tell about his promiscuity, exhibitionism and voyeurism would have hurt him, so in this case there was no solution except to disregard the neighbors, and live with her conscience. When, after five years, her first husband needed care at a nursing home, despite the fact that she had re-married, she visited him regularly making certain he had good care. The nursing home staff shunned her as well for divorcing that sweet deceptive man!

When a couple gets divorced, the children are affected by the tension. In addition, the parents who confide in their children cross the boundary of roles in the family.

One teenager observed his father mumble complaints about his mother. The teenager put his foot down, telling his father to cut it out, but by then he heard his father say a few derogatory things about the mother. "By mumbling you pretend that I should not hear what you are saying. All it does is, it makes me not want to get married" was the teenager's response.

When children ask their parents, who are about to get divorced, why they are getting divorced – the answer is: "We have problems and we've decided to get divorced." The children are not given details and the single response they should receive is: "Both of us love you and will continue to love you". The more you explain, the less they understand.

VIII
Step Parenting

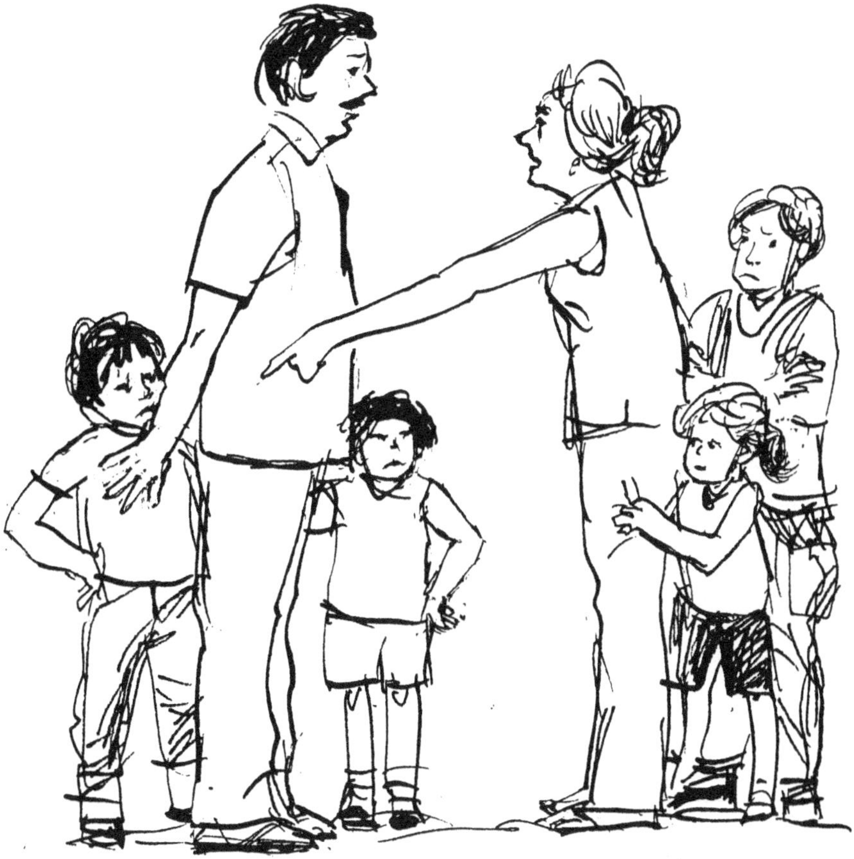

Step Parenting

Children are often unaware that they hurt their biological parent by rejecting their step parent, thereby turning the biological parent against the step parent. Children, with few exceptions, resent their biological parent for marrying a "stranger", but they resent the new step parent even more. This antagonistic relationship may exist no matter what age the parents and children are. Unpleasant discussions between the biological parent and the step parent are ignited when the step parent is mistreated by a step child, or when a step parent mistreats a step child. More often than not, it is the biological parent's fault for permitting his biological child to turn against the newly "acquired" step parent. When the biological parent shields his child from the step parent, it is overindulgence and it widens the gap. At the same time allowing that child to manipulate or act out repressed anger and frustration at his step parent is a form of indulgence.
Children who have been raised to "own" their parent, often cause acrimony between their biological parent and their step parent.

A woman with three children from a previous marriage married a man with two children from a previous marriage. The man got along with his step children, whereas the woman had major conflicts with her step children. The man tried his best to get everyone under the same roof to get along. The one major error he made was to badmouth his wife behind her back to his own family, namely, his sister and his parents. As a result, they demonstrated their dislike for his wife, shunning her and communicating their disapproval. The wife, in turn, complained to her husband about his children's behavior toward her, which caused more stress.

One father complained that his second wife was overly strict with his biological son from his first marriage and not strict enough with their biological children. "There are two sets of rules," he complained, that his wife was hypersensitive and negative when he wanted to do something fun with his biological son, yet when he wanted to do something fun with their biological children, she had no problem. When she was asked: "What is the hardest part of being a step parent?" she replied: "the spouse" and the fact that as the step parent, she is "one step removed."

While all this goes on between the biological parent and the step parent, the competition for that child's love between the two biological parents continues past their divorce, each trying to be nicer to their biological child, bending backwards to make sure the child has fun, fun, fun!

It is most often the biological parent's fault, when the step child and step parent don't get along. Feeling guilty for having re-married, the biological parent may try to "make it up" to his child, which is a form of over-indulgence. The biological parent is remiss in not laying down the law and instructing his biological child to behave properly toward the step parent!

A divorced man asked a divorced woman to marry him. She said she'd have to think about it. He then offered to take her and his fourteen year old biological son on vacation. As they approached his car, his son jumped into the front seat. The soon to be stepmother was relegated to the back seat for a long car ride. The boy's father said nothing to his son about his behavior. When they got back home, to add insult to injury, the boy blurted out: "I now know why I've been having headaches. It's seeing the two of you together all the time." The soon to be stepmother, having second thoughts right along, had a clear picture of what her life would be like after marriage, where she would be relegated to the "back seat".

IX

Psychoanalysis

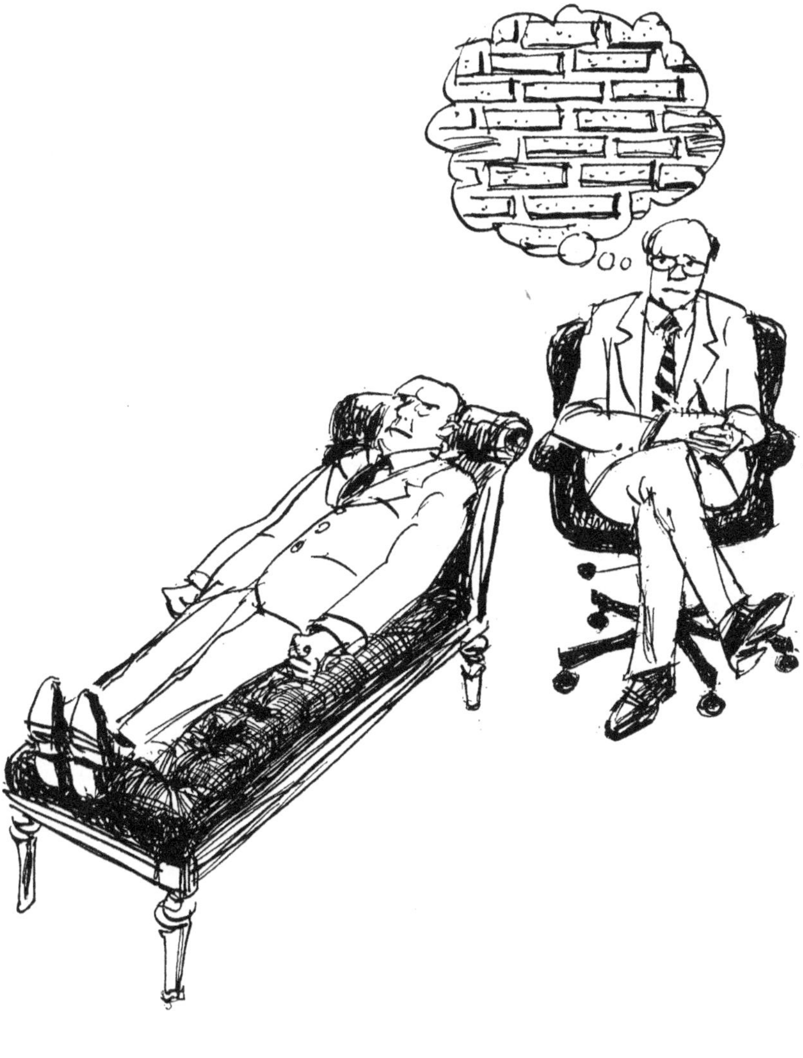

Psychoanalysis

The psychoanalytic journey is made up of two people engaged in a professional, emotionally explosive, intimate relationship where one does not want to say everything, the other does not want to hear everything, and yet, to achieve cure, both resistances must be resolved.

Psychoanalysis is thinking out loud. The therapist dealing with the "Enema Generation" (patients who resist talking freely, whose parents anticipated their every need) has to ask endless questions for the patient to keep talking.

The emotionally infantile patient soon learns that his needs are met only up to a point, and that he must learn to ask for what he wants and then he may not get what he asks for. Demands are analyzed and often remain ungratified, a painful process for both patient and analyst to endure. The analyst is not required to tell the patient everything, but he is expected to be truthful.

Mental hospitals are full of people who know why they are sick. Understanding does not cure nor resolve the patient's state of mind. Interpretations by the therapist do not clear up the problem. Getting to the root of the problem paints a clearer picture, but is nevertheless not useful in resolving the problem. It is the relationship between the patient and analyst – where the patient is able to say everything, which promotes resolution of problems via the transference (early feelings toward the parent, transferred unto the analyst).

When a problem is resolved over a long period of time, another, less toxic problem will likely replace it. When a problem is overcome (giving it up under pressure), a worse problem will likely replace it. Trying to erase all problems leaves an emotional cadaver, a dull and often medicated person.

People are often ashamed and hesitant to divulge having been prescribed antidepressants, being unaware of how prevalent it is.

In almost every family there is at least one person taking antidepressants.

"How did it make you feel?" is an ego-oriented, and therefore intrusive question, whereas "How did it make him feel?" does not involve the patient's ego. "Where was the restaurant?" is an object-oriented question – which deals with facts, not the patient's feelings and ego, and helps the patient talk.

Trying to get rid of a feeling is an impossible task. It's best to keep all feelings and develop new ones to counteract the undesirable feelings.

If a patient passes his therapist's advice to someone else, it may be as toxic as taking another person's medication, causing an "allergic" psychological reaction. Most patients have one foot out the door throughout the analytic treatment. If the analyst would not have to work so hard to keep patients in treatment, more could be accomplished, benefiting the patient.

A person's attitudes towards himself and others take years to be cultivated. It therefore takes a lengthy process to undo unhealthy attitudes. People wait and wait for the analyst to cure them. They don't realize that they must reach a point where they decide to change and change. Too often they want other people around them to change, and that's what they spend their sessions talking about.

Patients in analysis change but are often not accepted as having changed by their family and their community. A patient's treatment will be undermined if his home environment is destructive. Unable to have an arena in which to practice his newfound strength without being beaten down, the patient will regress and the treatment will fall into disarray.

The analyzed person has general self-awareness, speaks a "different language," and finds it difficult to relate to the unanalyzed. The well analyzed have the ability to say everything and to hear everything! When one person in a relationship is analyzed and the other is not, the relationship will undergo stress.

Resilience measures a person's emotional health. If he recovers from a narcissistic emotional injury (an insult) in ten minutes or so, he is emotionally healthy. If it takes him a couple of hours, it is a borderline case. If it takes him several hours, or if he brings up the problem again and again, he is emotionally unstable.

Unexpressed muted anger breeds depression. A depressed person induces in others concern which is eventually replaced by a desire to put him out of his misery. When a patient is angry at the analyst, yet expresses anger about someone else's behavior in the psychoanalytic session, it has little therapeutic value. Verbal anger directed at the analyst is therapeutic, providing the analyst accepts it without recrimination and the patient's complaints are not repeated.

Once transference develops in the psychoanalytic relationship, the patient is anchored in commitment and, unfortunately, some therapists are downright damaging, recommending family members cut off contact with each other, such as: "Stay away from your brother ...", which causes irreparable damage.

When selecting a mental health professional, particularly for young children, it is important to get good references and recommendations from the family physician. There are competent and incompetent professionals and workers in every profession and every field. There is a good plumber and a bad plumber, a good teacher and a poor teacher. When it comes to mental health professionals, many people seem to believe that just about all of them are competent.

Some examples: One psychoanalyst, to help her patient fall asleep, suggested she should imagine a grotesque fantasy, which had a lasting negative effect on the patient, who left treatment and entered treatment with a different therapist.

Regression, an inability to function, caused by irresponsible and destructive psychoanalytic treatment, could be irreversible, the damage lasting a lifetime. One psychoanalyst cut down a patient's appointments without warning, causing the patient to break down emotionally, leaving treatment and never recovering. The

patient, not yet immunized against the parent's toxicity, when prematurely experiencing the same toxic feelings from the analyst, will crumble, and the analyst's tools to reverse the patient's early psychological damage will be forfeited, the treatment coming to a sudden end.
The sicker the patient, the closer he is to his own unconscious mind, and thus, his assessment of the analyst's unconscious is often on target. This sensitivity made him susceptible to the parent's unexpressed feelings and later to the analyst's feelings.
Some children "absorb" their parent's emotional illness, thereby enabling the parent to act seemingly normal, their children carrying the "burden". "The unconscious mind knows everything."

The child who was adored by the parent in a one-to-one setting, while disliked in family situations, not infrequently will induce the same feelings in the analyst. The analyst's reaction toward that patient in family therapy may change from the one-to-one contact. Appearing helpless on the couch, the patient in the other settings, such as in group therapy may appear mean-spirited. The change in the analyst's countertransference (reaction to the patient's transference) may be experienced by the patient as a narcissistic injury (a painful, inconsolable, psychological injury accompanied by depression).

One woman told her therapist that when she was a little girl her mother took her places where men had sex with her. Her therapist not only believed it, where there was no way of knowing if it was true – the therapist anchored it into seeming "reality" by asking many questions and then instructing the woman to cut off all contact with her mother. When years later the mother was dying of cancer and asked to have her daughter visit her, the daughter refused, and then stayed away from the funeral, rejecting her father who had suffered a great loss.

If the mental health professional isn't talented, well trained and doesn't live by standards of decency, integrity and good morals, breaks up family relationships, encouraging the patient to talk about perverse memories, the patient will regress. It is never clear whether the "memories" actually occurred. It's not a question of disbelief. It's simply best to let the patient talk and the analyst withhold comment.

A couple had individual appointments with the same therapist – after which one partner told the other partner untruths about what she had told the therapist and what the therapist advised, causing the listening partner to believe it, not suspecting that they were lies. The patient's stories were intended to preserve the relationship between the partners, while making the therapist appear recklessly unethical, bringing their professional relationship with the therapist to an end.

A person dedicated to the psychoanalytic process, abiding by the contract and respecting the analyst, if confronted by an inquiring friend who intrudes and plays analyst and then ridicules the treatment, undermines the analyst's work, which may carelessly bring the treatment to an abrupt end. On the other hand, the one in treatment who cuts off the conversation and refuses to respond to any questions, will put the intruder in his place.
If the friend is permitted to play analyst and supervisor, not only will the treatment be jeopardized, but the well-being of the one in treatment will be tampered with. Too often people who need to be analyzed state: "I can talk to my friends."

Telling a patient that he is depressed will be tolerated, while labeling him "paranoid", "manic-depressive", "bi-polar" or "schizophrenic" can cause damage, for the diagnosis "sticks", which may spiral the patient further into a state of emotional despair. One patient repeated to everyone: "I'm mentally ill", practically wearing these words, unable to get out of the emotional "quick sand".

The narcissistic patient will enter into a rollercoaster relationship with the analyst, alternating between undying love and murderous hate. Being in the presence of a depressive, unforgiving narcissist is enough to make the analyst want to escape into a narcissistic countertransference where his self-preoccupation distracts him from destructive impulses toward the patient. The analyst whose emotional cobwebs have not been cleared in his own analysis, may have his problems entangle with those of the patient. Add to that an analyst who has a narcissistic spouse, and his level of immunity to the toxicity of the narcissistic patient is diminished. If the analyst's spouse is competing for his time – the analyst's judgment can be affected. The analyst will find it particularly difficult to work with severely derailed, narcissistic patients if his own family interactions are toxic.

Psychoanalytic Diagnostic Codes

Instead of using their time and their talents to find cures for illnesses, our society has "forced" physicians and mental health professionals to become entranced in figuring out medical diagnoses. There are over 100,000 diagnostic codes, with 1,000 codes changing each year. There are also 25,000 procedure codes which must be entered on the patient's insurance forms. Figuring out the correct diagnostic and procedure codes is time consuming for the doctor who must spend time looking up information in the 600 page CPT book.

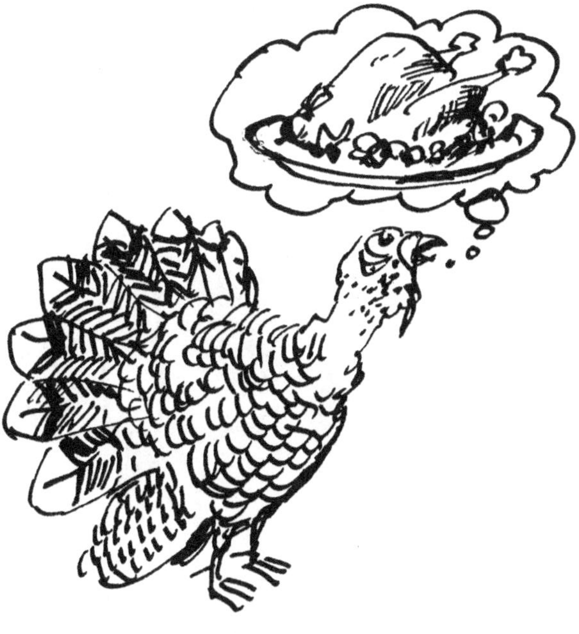

Acute Stress Disorder 308.3

This could be me next Thanksgiving!
Get that image out of my head! I'm stressed out!

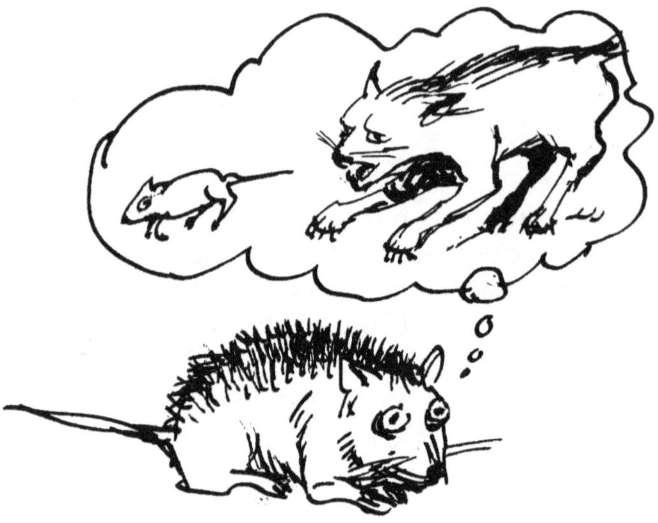

Post Traumatic Stress Disorder 309.81

I can't forget that scary cat chasing me!

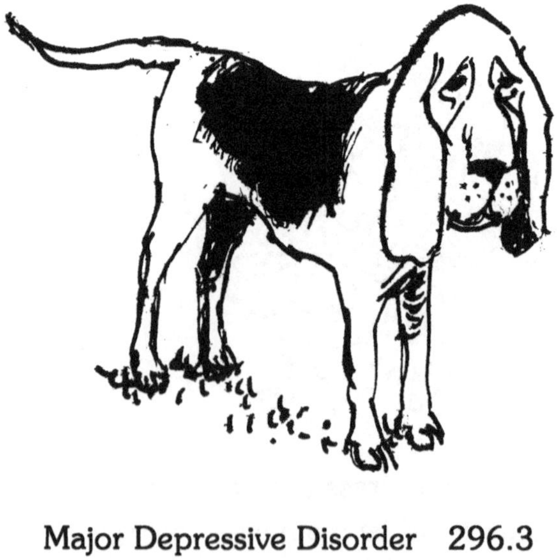

Major Depressive Disorder 296.3

I have no energy. I'm all alone. I'm not interested in life. Everything is wrong.

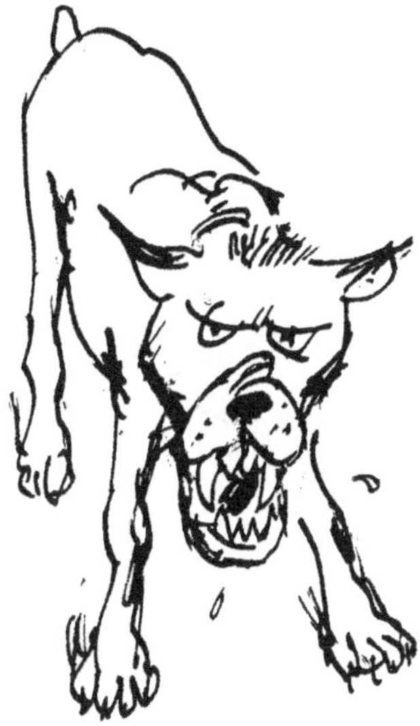

Intermittent Explosive Disorder 312.34

I'm going to scare you with my bark
and it won't be my fault! Woof!

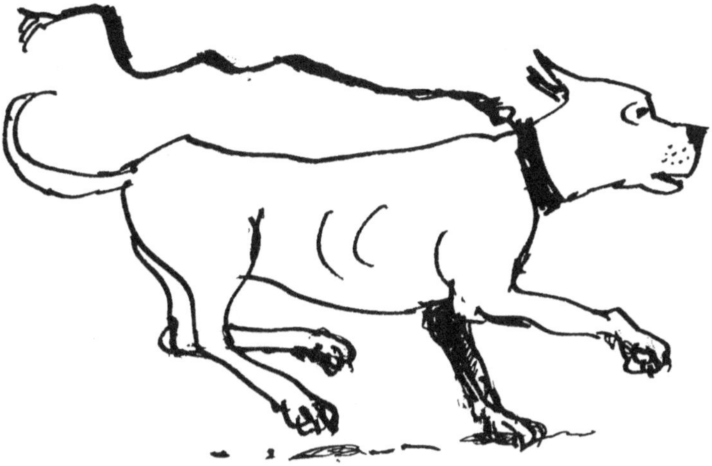

Panic Disorder 300.01

I can't stop these panic attacks. Here comes one;
I'm trying to get away;

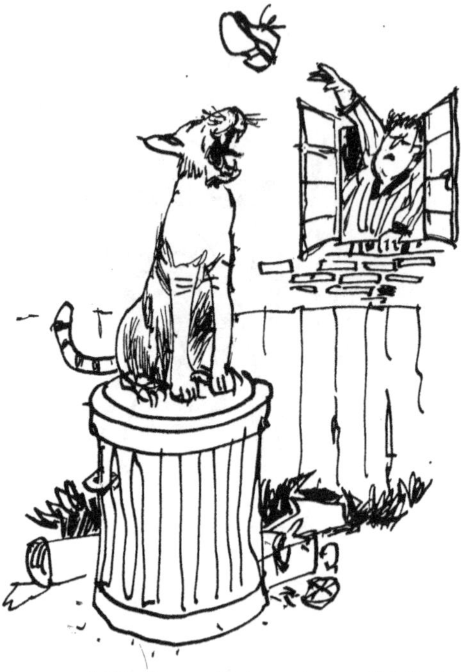

Oppositional Defiant Disorder 313.81

He thinks his shoe is going to silence me!
It provokes me to meow louder and louder and louder!

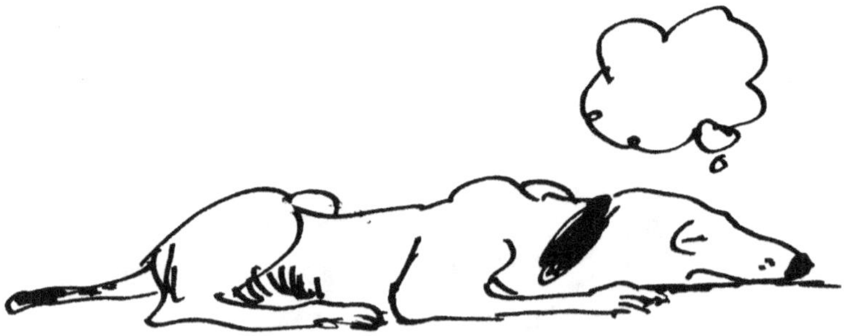

Narcolepsy 367.0

I sleep away the day. I can't stay awake!
Snore snore!

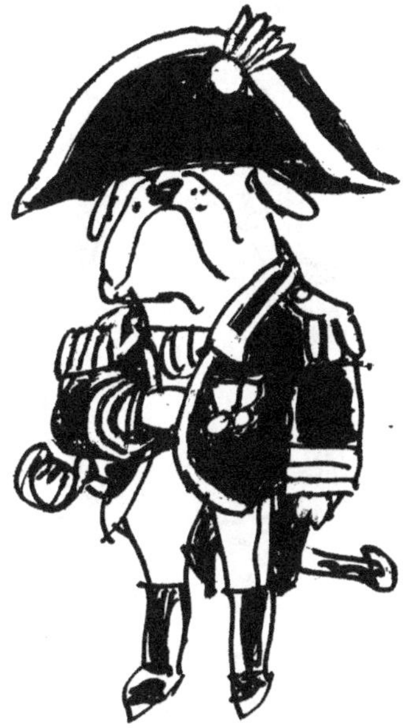

Delusional Disorder 291.1

I am Napoleon! If you think I'm a dog, you are wrong!

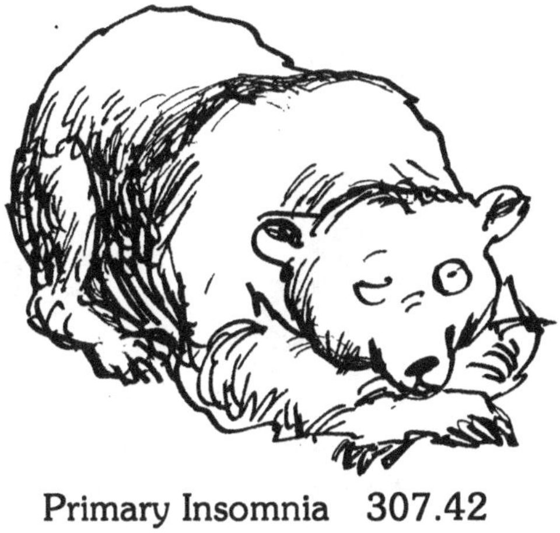

Primary Insomnia 307.42

I can't sleep. I am not going to function in daytime and get along in social situations. No way!

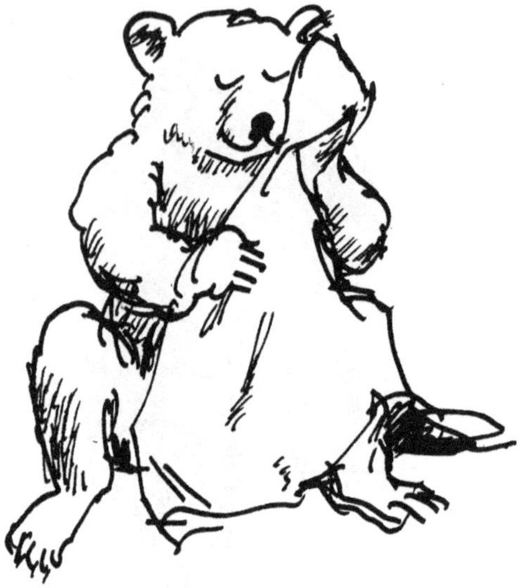

Separation Anxiety 309.21

I have a stomach ache and I need my mommy.
I want to sleep in her bed!
Mommy!

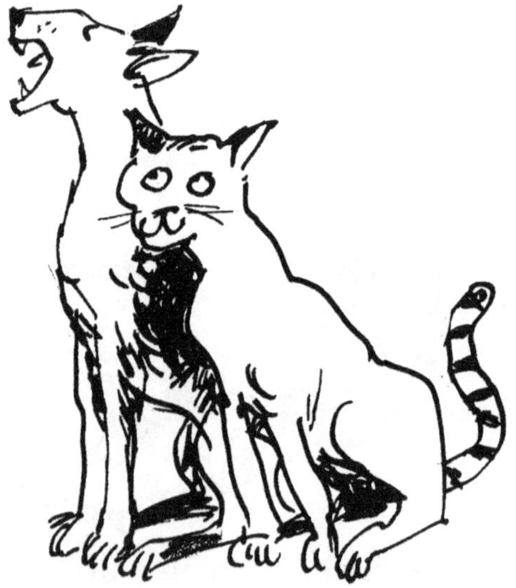

Hypoactive Sexual Desire Disorder 302.89

I'm sexually aroused and love rubbing
against a non-consenting dog.

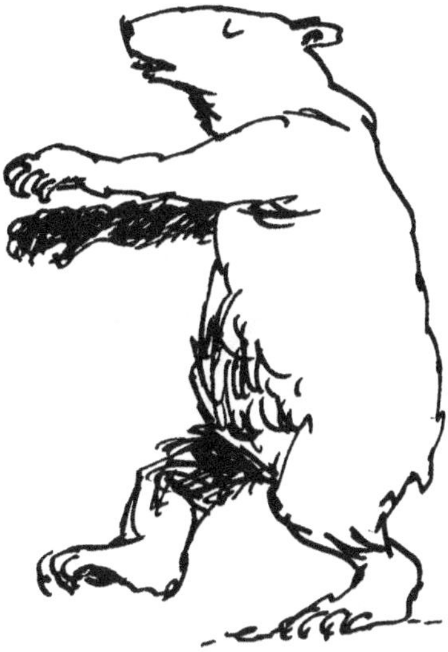

Sleepwalking Disorder 307.46

I screamed – got up and walked in my sleep.
No one can comfort me. I'm sweaty and out of it!

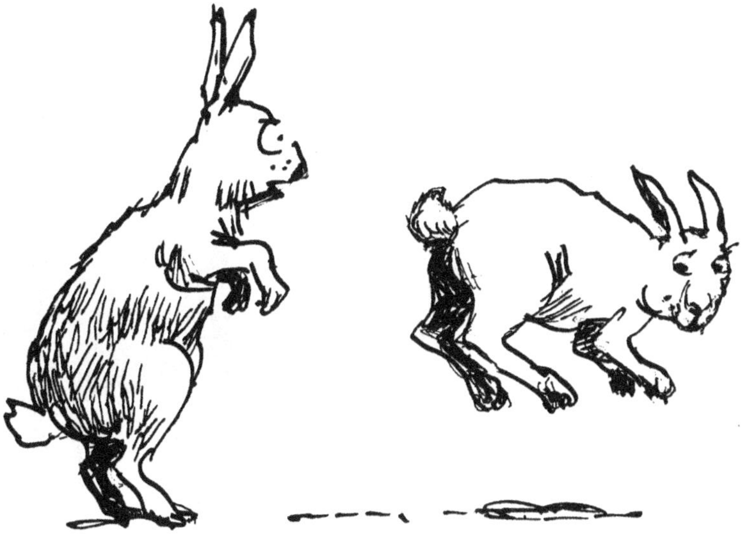

Sexual Aversion Disorder 302.79

No! No! I said no! Go away!
No sex! No! Don't touch me!

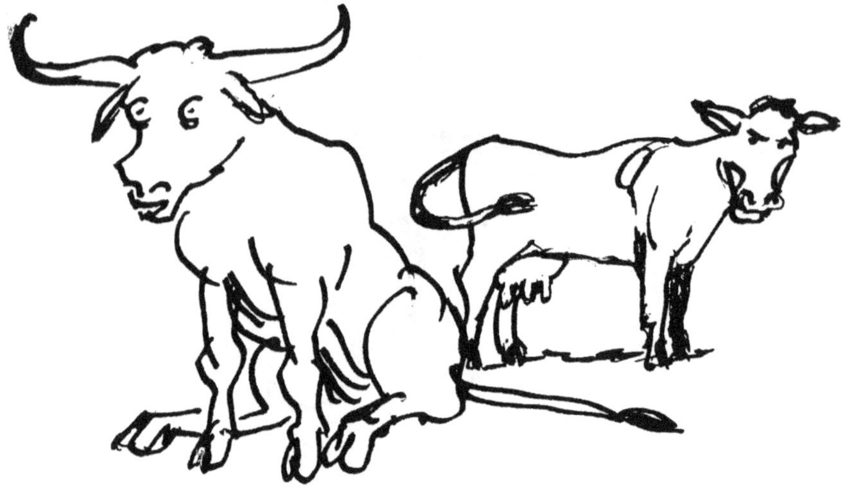

Male Erectile Disorder 302.72

Don't look so annoyed, cow! I can't help that I'm impotent! Moo!

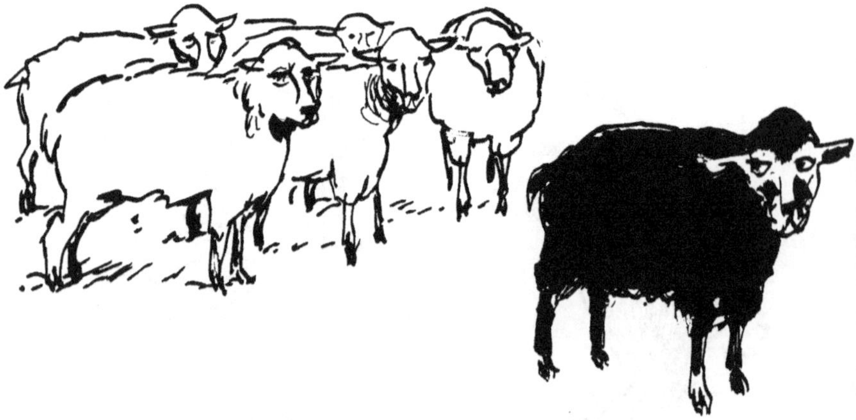

Social Phobia 300.23

I'm a black sheep. I'm mocked and humiliated!

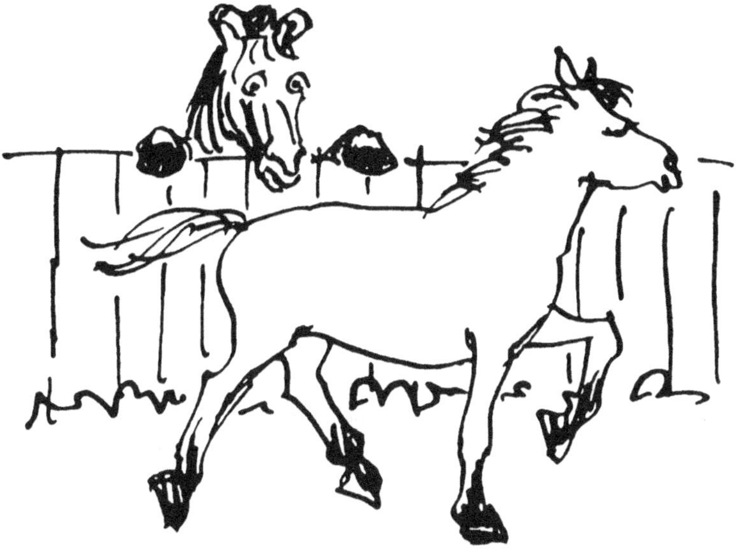

Voyeurism 302.82

I'm observing an unsuspecting sexy horse! Wow!

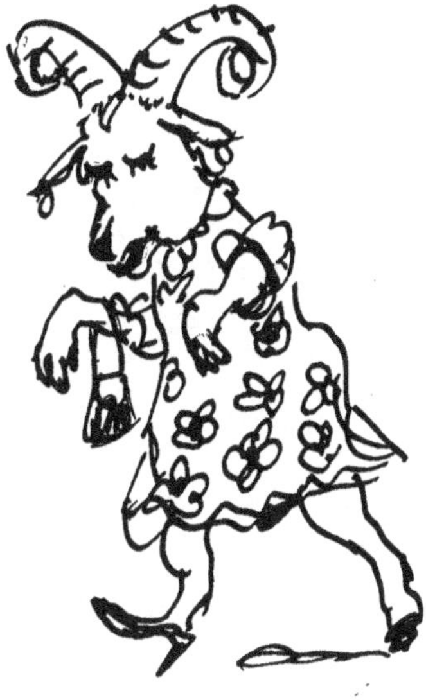

Transvestite Fetishism 302.3

I cross-dress to look like a pretty female,
even though I am a heterosexual male.
Oh! And these fingernails!

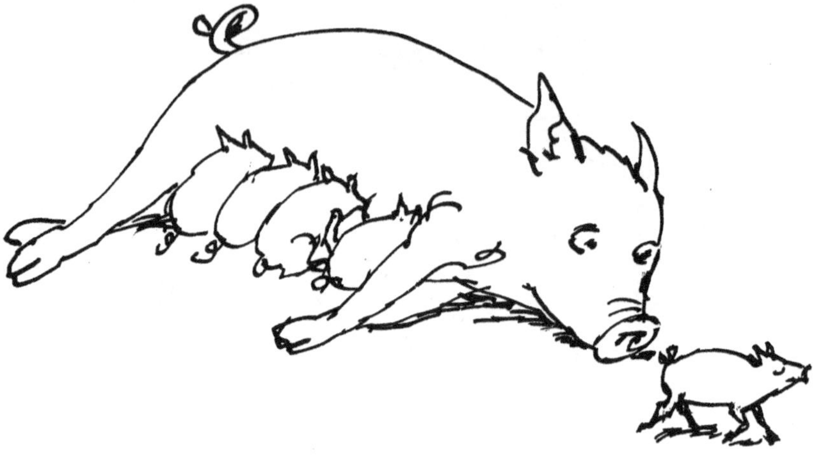

Feeding Disorder, Infancy or Children 307.59

I can't eat like a pig!
I am a malnourished baby pig
because Mommy has too many other babies.
There's no room for me!

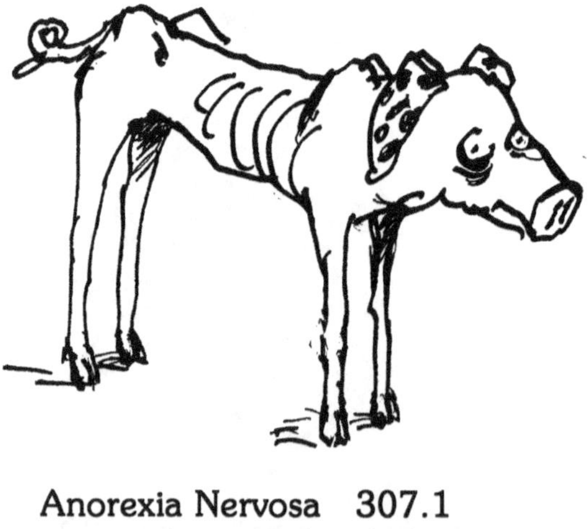

Anorexia Nervosa 307.1

I'm embarrassed to eat in public!
I'm so scared of gaining weight!
I get on the scale every hour.
I look in the mirror and see fat!

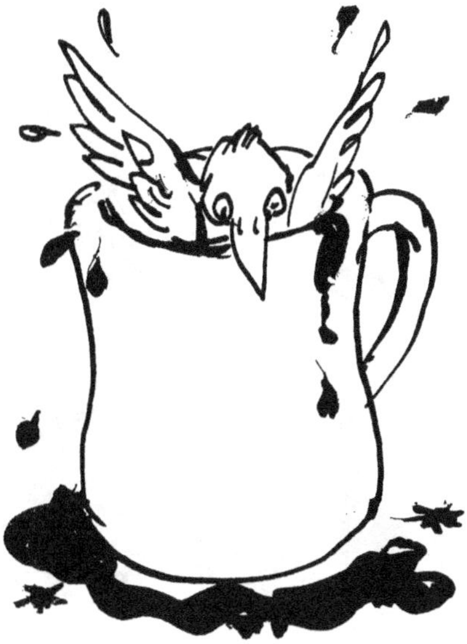

Caffeine Intoxication 305.90

This coffee is yummy, but it makes me hyper,
restless and twitchy!
Twitch twitch!

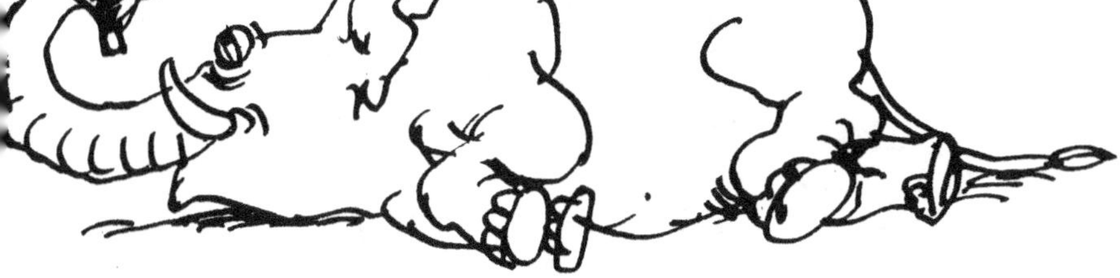

Alcohol Withdrawal 291.8

My bottle is empty!
My heart beats fast and I'm nauseous! Yuk!

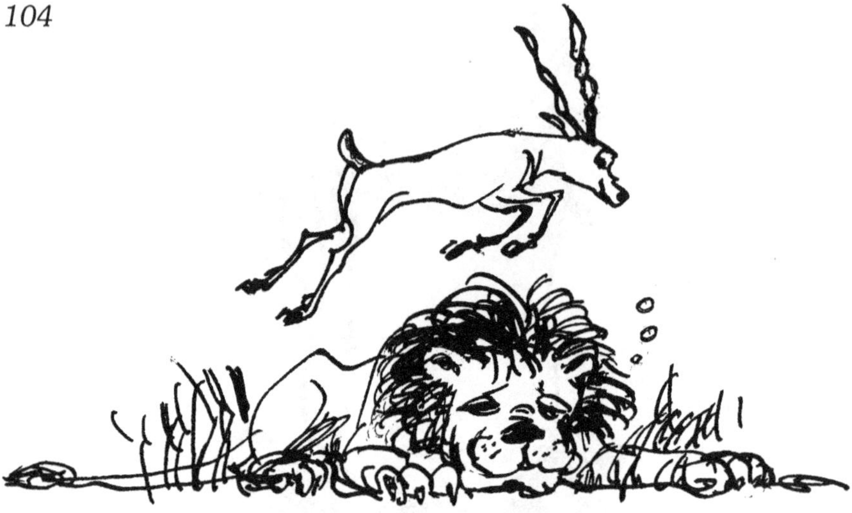

Alcohol Intoxication 303.00

I'm drunk! I'm in a stupor from alcohol!
I imagine a deer flying over me!

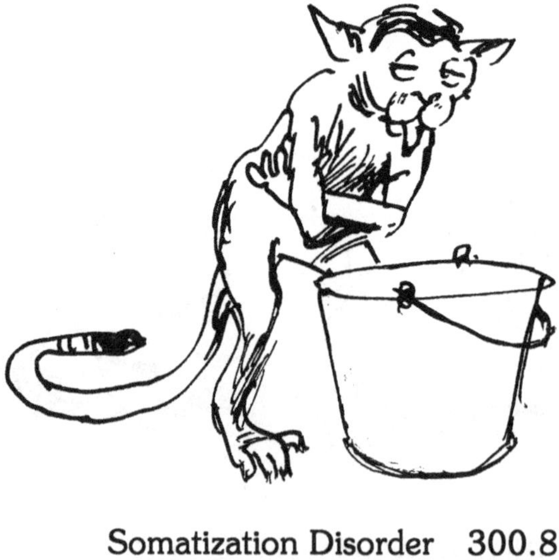

Somatization Disorder 300.81

My neck, back and joints hurt!
I'm nauseous and vomiting! I hate sex!

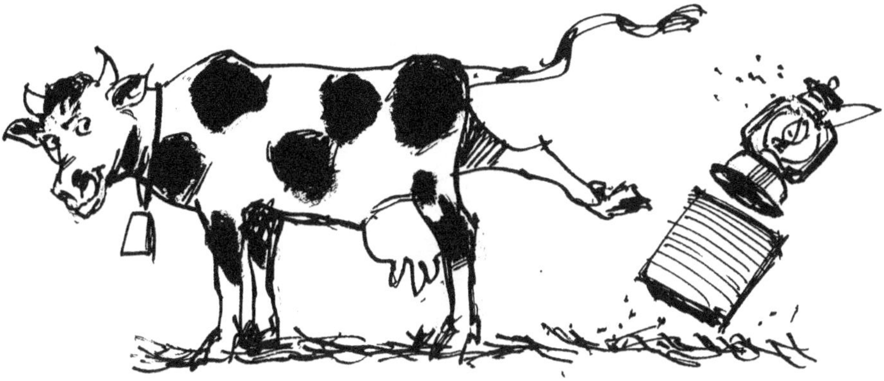

Pyromania 312.33

Deliberately setting fires releases my tensions, and it's great fun!

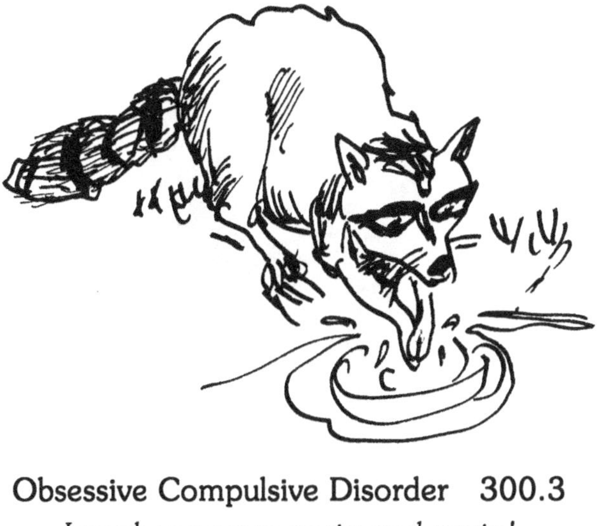

Obsessive Compulsive Disorder 300.3

I wash my paws again and again!
I hope germs won't get me!
I repeat words and prayers over and over to keep away the demons!

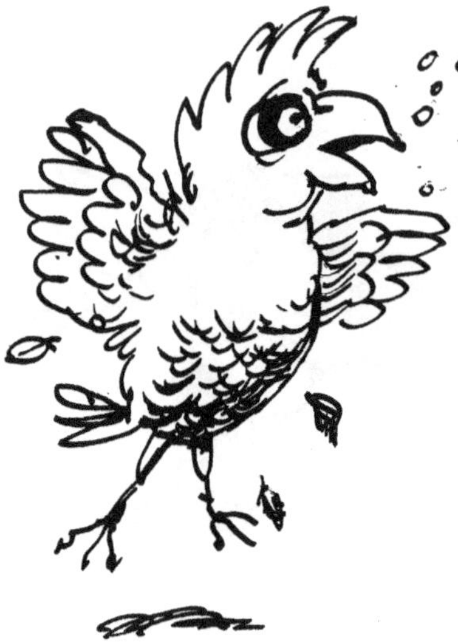

Chronic Motor-Vocal Tic Disorder 307.22

I make sudden rapid motions and odd sounds.
I wonder why no one wants to be around me!

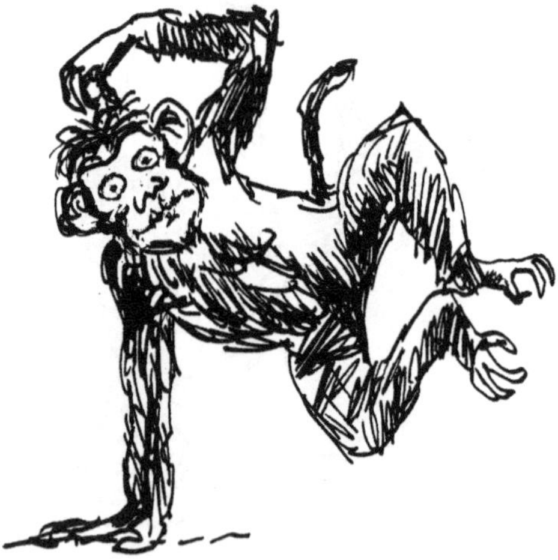

Catatonic Type 295.20

I'll get into bizarre, rigid postures.
If you don't like it, lump it.
I don't obey any instructions, except my own.

X

Sexuality

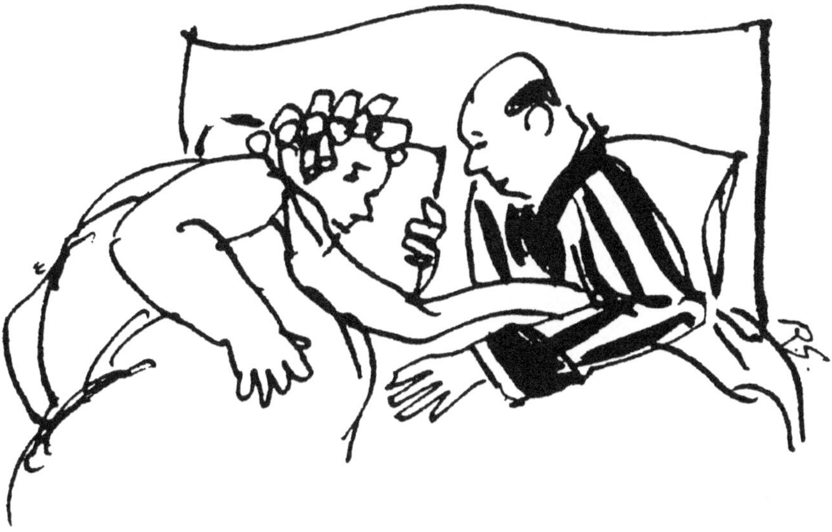

Sexuality

When a person reports "early memories" of being molested and the listener shows great interest by asking endless questions, e.g.: "How many times did it happen?", "Where was your mother?", "Who did you tell it to?" etc., the "memory" is encouraged and often embellished. It is best to listen in silence. If, on the other hand, a child reports ongoing sexual contact, the listener immediately informs the parents and the law enforcement.

A child permitted to visit his parents' bedroom at night (sometimes getting into their bed) is harmful to all concerned, interfering in the parents' private relationship. Contrary to what parents often believe, a child feels more secure if returned to his own bed, rather than being permitted to remain in his parents' bed. Crying himself to sleep is far less harmful than sharing the bed with his parents. Sleeping in a separate bed in his parents' bedroom causes the child to become an unhealthy instrument in his parents' relationship, in the process damaging himself as well.

Over-indulging children inadvertently gives them the "right", as they grow up, to do all kinds of things in life which are negative. In marriage, they are unfaithful and may turn to exhibitionism and voyeurism. The married man may flirt with women, insulting his wife in several ways: the wife appears to these women as a loser and seemingly unimportant to her husband, so they feel sorry for her, for they are convinced that her man would rather be with them!
On the other hand, parents who are disciplinarian, who set limits – "you can't do this, it's not allowed!" – will bring up children who, as adults, will know and respect boundaries of decency and faithfulness in marriage.

Surprising as it may seem, a child does not require constant reassurance that the parents love him. All physical contact arouses some sexual feelings, regardless of whether the contact is pleasurable (hugging, kissing and tickling) or painful (hitting, slapping). Tickling or rubbing a child's extremities is seductive. Relatives have no business giving a child a hug or asking for a hug, or telling the child to hug someone else, unless the child thinks of it himself. An adult who tells a child: "Go kiss your grandmother," "Give your uncle a hug," "Come over here and give me a hug" seem well intentioned, but nevertheless are improper. Hugging a child or directing the child to hug or kiss someone else is intruding into his right to privacy! Shaking hands is an acceptable greeting for both children and adults.

A parent who sits on the couch with his arm around his teenager, (particularly a parent of the opposite sex) makes a statement of physical ownership. Parents who hug their children in public believing that they communicate to onlookers: "I love my children so much!" turn onlookers into uncomfortable voyeurs. At religious services, it is particularly noticeable when parents physically embrace their offspring – some having already reached puberty. The parents mean well, but are, nevertheless, destructive.

Counselors participating in the filming of misbehaved children for a television show, claimed that the children were not harmed by the experience because they were "fundamentally secure". Interesting words that mean nothing! Infringing on a child's right to privacy is exhibitionistic, while attracting a voyeuristic audience.

When discussing sex, the father is the one that should talk to his son and the mother to her daughter. It's inappropriate, uncomfortable and sexually stimulating when the daughter speaks to her father and the son to his mother.

A twelve year old girl pointed to a mirror and exclaimed: "There's a man in the shower!" In the mirror she saw the hazy outline of a paunch and quite a bit more behind the foggy shower stall. "Oh, oh no. That's, that's just my dad. No big deal. He always showers with the door open 'cause the fan is broken." Harmless as it may seem, it is a mistake to bathe with the door open or to bathe children together, regardless of their age or sex, since curiosity and a desire to touch each other's genitals may be aroused. Spectators (except the parent in charge) are virtually voyeurs and should not be allowed in the bathroom. Parental modesty is required for children to grow up sexually adjusted. A sexual perversion is not a one time "mistake" and is not easily cured.

In an open eating cafeteria, a seated obese woman put her foot on the chair in front of her, bent her knee and placed her two year old boy on her leg, took out her breast, and pointed the nipple at him, who immediately grabbed it with his mouth and started to suck. The whole place was astounded at her lack of privacy. Seeing several mothers with their young children seated at the same table, one disapproving older woman walked over and said to the nursing mother: "You are out of line," to which the mother did not respond while continuing to nurse.

When a newborn vomits after nursing and is then frequently given the second breast, he is over-indulged. Should that happen daily, the parent better prepare to take care of the "baby" (who whimpers: "Mommy is delicious") until the last day of his life.

A middle aged couple hugged, caressed, kissed and touched each other improperly on the roof of a parking garage, where people gathered to view a 4th of July fireworks display. The exhibitionistic display made parents and children on that roof uncomfortable.

It's not having been "abused" in childhood which causes sexual perversions later in life. It's overindulgence!!!

In all relationships there are written, and unwritten "contracts". If a contract is broken, the relationship is at risk until a new contract (agreement) is established and defined. Most prominently, overgratification communicates to the child, as he grows up, that everything is up for grabs including sexual infidelity, exhibitionism and voyeurism.

"I am the parent. I make the rules, you are the child, you obey them," is a contract that seems simple. It is not. It's a difficult contract for parents to adhere to, particularly because the long term consequences don't seem as ominous as they can be. When the parent permits the child to run the show, the child disregards the contracts within his family. When grown up, he will not adhere to the marriage vows, venturing outside the marital relationship for sexual gratification. He may pay bills late, or not at all, leading to bankruptcy or collection agencies knocking at his door. He may sleep late when he should be at work and family members are afraid to wake him up. His single wish is seeking pleasure, while the marital contract is disregarded and scoffed at. Having learned, as a child, that contracts were made to be broken, as an adult he will overspend, overeat and eat the wrong foods. Since there were no consequences to contend with when his parents permitted him to cajole them into breaking the parent-child contract, he had free reign, which lasts a lifetime. Once the parent decides to discipline that teenager for the first time, it becomes a useless confrontation – where the parent has no power. Parents who claim that their offspring have reached adulthood and should be responsible for their own actions, fail to take responsibility for the part they played in overindulging their children who had grown into out-of-control adults.

A father had sex with his daughter beginning when she was thirteen. By the age of twenty two she had given birth to a baby who she tossed to his death, out the window. A year later, she once again conceived her father's child, making him both the father and grandfather of the infant whom she proceeded to toss out the window once more. The father of the two dead babies, along with <u>his</u> parents should be held accountable for the mayhem!

XI
Physical Health

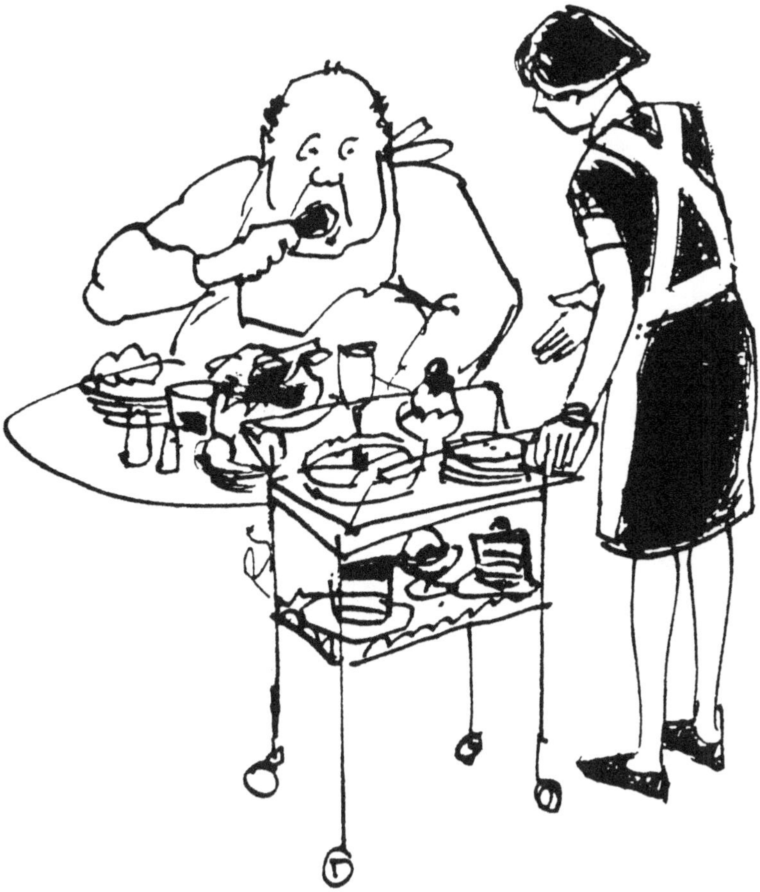

Physical Health

1. Avoiding Dangers

Flaxseed

In 3500 BC the Egyptians were making their papyrus (the paper on which they wrote) from “flax” and they had a lot of flax seed left over which they fed to their sheep, pigs and cattle. All the animals died. No one knows why they died but it might have been from the fatty acid called alpha linolenic acid in flax seed oil. A similar fatty acid called gamma linolenic acid is essential for making myelin that covers the nerves in the brain. With large amounts of flax seed oil being consumed and circulating through the body in the blood stream, flax seed oil may be replacing the gamma linolenic acid surrounding the nerves which would cause the nerves to die. In 5 to 10 years from now there might be a large number of people dying from damaged brains.

Flax seed and flax seed oil are being widely advertised to help people prevent hardening of the arteries and heart attacks. It is recommended because it has a large amount of an omega-3 fatty acid in it but it is not the same omega-3 fatty acid that the body makes and the body cannot convert the flax seed fatty acid into the kind of omega-3 fatty acid that is essential for making the brain work. Fish oils that are successful in preventing heart attacks also contain large amounts of an omega-3 fatty acid, but it is not the same one that is in flax seed oil. There is a big chemical difference between the omega-3 fatty acid in fish oil and the omega-3 fatty acid in flax seed oil. No experiments have ever been done that show that flax seed oil helps people in any way.

Omega-3 Fatty Acids

The Omega-3 fatty acids that help prevent heart attacks are found only in ocean-raised fish. Krill, shrimp-like crustaceans that feed on the plant-like plankton, make the omega-3 fatty acids. Krill do not live in fish ponds. If salmon are trapped in Norwegian fjords and fenced-off from the ocean and fed with food grown on a farm, those salmon would have fat but it would not have the omega-3 fatty acid that is therapeutic and comes from krill. Salmon raised in ponds on land and fed from land grown crops would also not have any of the therapeutic omega-3 fatty acids.

Salmon that live in the ocean do not eat krill themselves but eat the smaller fish that eat the krill. Small fish eat the krill and store the omega-3 fatty acids in their bodies. These small fish are eaten by larger fish such as salmon and they too store the omega-3 fatty acids.

Peanuts

Aflatoxin is a chemical that is made by a fungus that lives on the hulls of peanuts. It is a poisonous chemical that causes cancer of the liver. The Food and Drug Administration (FDA) has put a strict limit on the amount of aflatoxin that may be present in commercial peanut butter. There is no limit on the amount of aflatoxin there is in peanuts and peanut butter sold in health food stores. The FDA has no jurisdiction over herbs and foods sold in stores.

In addition to the danger of aflatoxin, peanuts are the best way to cause hardening of the arteries and heart attacks in monkeys. All the researchers who study coronary artery disease in monkeys, feed them peanuts to cause coronary disease. If monkeys eat their natural food they do not get hardening of the arteries and heart attacks but if they eat peanuts they do. The metabolism of people is not too different from that of monkeys. No studies have been done on the effect of peanuts on people, because nobody wants to design an experiment that shows that peanuts kill people. Not all nuts are dangerous. Some nuts are definitely beneficial.

Walnuts and Brazil Nuts

To demonstrate that beneficial effects can be caused by some nuts, a controlled study was done with walnuts. People were randomly assigned to one of 2 groups. One group had to eat 35 walnuts a day and the other group was forbidden to eat any nuts. The group eating walnuts had fewer heart attacks than those who did not. What made walnuts beneficial is probably gamma linolenic acid, an essential fatty acid that is required for making the myelin sheath around the nerves in the brain.

12% of the fatty acids in walnuts are gamma linolenic and 46% of the fatty acids in Brazil nuts are gamma linolenic. Brazil nuts and Walnuts increase the amount of HDL (*H*igh *D*ensity *L*ipoprotein) in the blood. HDL cholesterol is the good cholesterol.

Pistachios

The high oleic content in Pistachios makes it look good as a source of monounsaturated fat. But pistachios are dry roasted, which makes it like a dangerous saturated fat. Walnuts and Brazil nuts are not roasted, so they increase the good HDL cholesterol.

Green Potatoes

Eating the green skin of a potato can be dangerous. The green color is a signal that glycoalkaloid is being made. 90% of glycoalkaloid is stored in the potato skin which can kill one if too much is eaten and is not influenced by cooking, frying, boiling, baking or steaming. The presence of inflammatory bowel disease is highest in countries where fried potato consumption is the highest. When a potato is dug out of the ground it is grey or brown. If allowed to be at room temperature and exposed to sunlight, the skin around the stem will become green. The green color is due to the synthesis of chlorophyll, which in itself is harmless, but glycoalkaloid is made at the same time as chlorophyll.

Grapefruit

A 32 year old mother of two was found dead on the floor of her parents' bathroom in Florida where her parents owned a grapefruit farm. The cause of death was not known until 3 years later, when it was clear that she had died of ventricular fibrillation of the heart due to drinking grapefruit juice while taking Seldane, a medicine used for allergies. The Seldane concentration in her body became higher and higher as a result of drinking grapefruit juice, until it was 20 times as high as normal and high enough to damage the heart and make it beat in a deadly irregular way that resulted in its stopping.
There are computer programs that a physician can use to check drug to drug interactions but they do not automatically check on all the drugs the patient is taking.

Mercury and Fish

Eating a lot of large fish, such as sword fish, tuna, shark, etc. may cause mild mercury poisoning. There is mercury in the ocean water and it is incorporated into a plant (plankton) which is eaten by krill, a shrimp-like crustacean which is then eaten by small fish which are eaten by large fish and the large fish are eaten by still larger fish.

The bigger the fish the more smaller fish it has eaten and therefore the more mercury it will contain. Salmon doesn't stay out in the ocean for more than 3 years and hence contains very little mercury. The fish oil and meat of the salmon is safe. Mercury is never attached to fish oil. If the fish has been raised in a fish pond, that fish contains no mercury. If there is any question about mercury, a sample of a person's blood will show if there is too much mercury in the blood. If there is mercury in the blood, one can get rid of it by taking dimercaprol.

Egg Yolk

Egg yolk is bad for people who have or have had a family history of hardening of the arteries, stroke, heart attack, angina, or who have an elevated cholesterol level. Hardening of the arteries is rare in people who have a total cholesterol measurement below 150 mg/dl (milligram per deci-liter) or an LDL (*L*ow *D*ensity *L*ipoprotein) cholesterol level below 70 mg/dl. The lower the total cholesterol or the lower the LDL cholesterol is, the less likely one will have hardening of the arteries. Egg yolk contains 1480 mg of cholesterol per 100 gm, which is more cholesterol than in any other food. The next most concentrated food source of cholesterol is chicken liver at 486 mg/100 gm.

The cholesterol in the body is recycled. The liver makes cholesterol. This and any cholesterol that was absorbed from food is excreted by the liver in the bile that is emptied into the small intestine. A large part of this bile excreted cholesterol is reabsorbed. When eating egg yolk, that cholesterol will go around and around and be excreted into the bile, then reabsorbed into the small intestine. It will be some time before the cholesterol from the egg yolk disappears. The extra cholesterol increases the risk of a heart attack.

It is well to remember that all vegetables, fruits and plant seeds have no cholesterol in them, since the cells in plants use cellulose for the cell membrane instead of cholesterol.

Vitamin A

One needs to be careful about taking vitamin A. It can be lethal. Arctic explorers trying to be the first to get to the North Pole in 1902 killed a white Arctic Snow Bear, cooked it and ate the liver which is very rich in Vitamin A. They all died of Vitamin A poisoning. The usual dose in over-the-counter multi-vitamins is 5000 units. This is the proper daily dose. 10,000 is more than one can use. 50,000 units is dangerous.

2. Advanced Medical Treatments

Ice Water Enema

Fever over 105° F in an adult must be lowered rapidly. If lowering is not done rapidly the temperature may rise to 107° F or 108° F. If the temperature stays there, brain damage occurs. Current treatments consist of cold blankets which take 2 or 3 hours to get the temperature down to 102° F or 103° F. This is not good enough.

The answer is an ice water enema. Two quarts of water cooled with ice given in 2 to 3 minutes gives fast relief. Blood flowing through the walls of the colon is not slowed down by ice cold water the way it is when using cold blankets. The total amount of blood in the body is 7 quarts. The heart pumps 6 quarts of blood a minute. At the end of 3 minutes the blood temperature would be lowered by 18° (if it was not being warmed by other parts of the body).

An ice water enema is not uncomfortable. There are no nerves in the walls of the colon that can detect whether the walls are cold or not. Also, the blood vessels in the colon do not constrict in the presence of cold water. All the blood vessels in the skin do constrict.

One patient with advanced cancer developed a temperature of 109° F. Repeated enemas of ice cold water in the colon caused the temperature to drop to 103° F in fifteen minutes.

Diagnosis of strep throat

Ten percent of the population in the United States have beta hemolytic streptococci growing in back of their throats. The streptococci do not stay there for more than 2 or 3 months because they cannot compete with the other bacteria growing in the throat.

People who are streptococci carriers seldom know that they are carriers transmitting the germ to other people during a conversation or from a cough etc.
The carrier might get a viral infection with a sore throat, fever and positive strep culture (yet it is not a streptococcal infection), and frequently have prescribed antibiotics when not necessary and children may be kept out of school. The sore throat and fever are not due to the streptococci which have been there for weeks or months. The symptoms are due to the viruses.
If there is a true streptococcal infection there is a rise in the blood's antibodies against streptococcus. If the body is fighting to kill the streptococci it makes antibodies against the protein S in the wall of the streptococcus. If it is a viral infection there will be no rise in antibodies against protein S.

A streptococcal infection is characterized by distinctive symptoms: a marked fever of 101°F or more at the onset, tenderness and enlargement of the lymph node just under the angle of the jaw. A bright red spot on the pharynx or a bright redness over all the pharynx is a sign of streptococcal infection. A streptococcal infection lasts less than 6 days without any treatment. An infection that lasts 6 days or more has less than one chance in a thousand of being a streptococcal infection.

If a person has a streptococcal infection and spontaneously recovers without antibiotics it is still worthwhile to give that patient penicillin as long as it is 15 days or less since the start of the infection. A 10 day course of 500 mg of penicillin 4 times a day is enough to prevent heart damage. If untreated, one person in 50, who had a strep infection, will get heart damage.

Going to Sleep

People who wake up at night to go to the bathroom and can not get back to sleep could use a simple remedy of eating or drinking one or two cups of something hot. The rationale behind it is: If the stomach is very hot the body will shunt blood from the brain to the stomach to cool the stomach down. If food is being digested, it requires energy and more blood flow is needed in the intestine. With more blood going to the stomach and less to the brain it is easier to go to sleep.

Muscle Cramps

Most muscle cramps come from a lack of sufficient potassium within the muscle cells. Massaging, heating, and stretching the involved muscle gives immediate relief. But the pain might return in a few minutes or a few hours. The way to prevent the cramps is to increase the potassium concentration within the cells. This only requires a very small increase in potassium concentration. The easiest and fastest way of doing this is to swallow some potassium chloride.

Potassium chloride is available as a powder which is sold in supermarkets under a variety of names, such as "Salt Substitute", "No Salt", or "Nu Salt". Norton's Salt Substitute contains 50% potassium chloride. The other 50% are chemicals to make the contents of the Salt Substitute more palatable. The container weighs 88 gm (~3 oz.) which is enough for 74 servings. One serving is ¼ of a teaspoon of the powder.

Potassium chloride is also available as tablets. The potassium chloride powder can not be taken as such. It must be diluted. The powder can be sprinkled over a food such as mashed potatoes or it can be dissolved in 2 or 3 teaspoons of a liquid such as orange juice, prune juice, vegetable juice, etc. If the concentrated potassium chloride is swallowed undiluted it could damage the walls of the esophagus, stomach and intestine.

When treating muscle cramps, take ¼ teaspoon of potassium chloride. If this does not work in 15 minutes, take a second dose. If the cramp persists repeat the ¼ of a teaspoon 2 more times at 30 minute intervals. If the cramp still persists, treat with heat, stretching, and massage. If this doesn't work, seek medical care. More than 4 doses in 90 minutes could be dangerous.

Bananas contain a lot of potassium and are often recommended as a substitute for potassium chloride. This does not work because the potassium in bananas is attached to an organic acid. Organic acids are destroyed by the body and replaced by potassium hydroxide which is an alkali. The kidneys get rid of excess alkalis in the blood by excreting potassium hydroxide in the urine.

Heel Spur

Heel spur pain is pain on the bottom of the heel, where the tendon attaches to the front of the heel bone. When one puts pressure on this point it hurts. The pain begins when one accidentally falls forward while lifting something heavy and most of one's weight is on that foot. The trauma causes the tendon to pull partially away from the heel. The body heals the tear by laying down bone. The process of laying down new bone takes 4 – 6 weeks. Putting pressure on the heel before it completely heals causes pain. With pain, one tends to walk on the front of the foot. This stretches the tendon from front to back and may pull the tendon further away from the heel. Healing and tearing goes on for a long time and as more bone is made the spur gets longer and longer. This can be prevented by taking pressure off the heel.

Take a piece of ½ inch thick woolen felt and cut out a piece that fits in the heel portion of the shoe and is about 6 – 7 cm long. With one thumb put pressure on the bottom of the heel until you find the spot that is tender. Then cut a hole in the felt where this sore spot is. Put the felt with a hole in it into the shoe. Put the shoe on and then stand up and put all of your weight on the heel. If that hurts, change the size or location of the hole until full weight on the heel does not cause pain. Use that shoe all the time or make more pads for any shoes that you do use. Then whenever you walk you feel no pain and now pay no attention to the heel. There is no need to walk on the ball of the foot and the tendon remains firmly attached to the heel bone. After 2 or 3 months, try walking without the pad in the shoe. If it hurts a bit use the pad for another month.

Underarm Odor

People try to control under arm odor by plugging up the ducts of the sebaceous glands. However, pressure builds up inside the glands which sooner or later forces the plug out and the odor comes out.

The cause of the odor is anaerobic bacteria growing on the sebum in the sebaceous gland. Anaerobic bacteria do not require oxygen to grow, they are easily destroyed by 1% clindamycin solution. To get rid of the odor, apply a 1% clindamycin solution to the underarm area for 10 continuous days (most antibiotics, like penicillin, can not kill anaerobes). Thereafter, apply clindamycin once a week. If the odor returns, apply 1% clindamycin daily for a week.

On Being Thirsty

There are two ways in which one can get thirsty: One way is by losing too much salt and the other is by losing too much water. One can lose too much salt by having diarrhea or vomiting, or by following a rigid salt-free diet. One can lose too much water by working in a hot environment and sweating a lot and not drinking enough water.

In the salt-loss case: Every time one drinks water the kidney senses that the concentration of salt in the blood is too low and that adding water will make the concentration of salt even lower, so the kidney gets rid of the extra water by putting it out in urine. The brain senses that the volume of blood needs to be increased and that is why one feels thirsty. The way to relieve this kind of thirst is to drink salty soup. The kidney will keep that water because it has salt in it.

In the water-loss case: The relief of thirst is simply drinking water. If one is working hard and sweating for a long time and not drinking any water, one will feel thirsty after a while. One will have lost volume from the circulatory system, i.e. water but not salt. Now the water one drinks stays in the body since the kidney recognizes that the concentration of salt is too high and adding water will lower the concentration. One will stay thirsty until one drinks enough water to bring the salt concentration down to normal. There will not be any excess urination.

Burning on Urination

When a woman gets a urinary infection it is usually very painful to urinate. This is because the wall of the bladder is raw and inflamed and the urine is usually acidic. If one pours acid on a cut or an open burn it hurts. Half a teaspoon of baking soda dissolved in water or prune juice, peach juice, etc. will change the urine from acidic to alkaline, and urination will be comfortable while waiting for antibiotics to cure the infection.

Preventing Wound Odors

Wounds that have been open for weeks or months, e.g. cancer, sometimes generate an unpleasant odor. This odor can be prevented by washing the wound with 10% lactose and then sprinkling the wound with the powder that is used for making yogurt. Lactose is the name for milk sugar. Lactose and yogurt powder can both be obtained over the internet. 10% is the concentration that is compatible with the tissues in the body. It is equivalent to the 5% glucose solution that is given intravenously. The powder for making yogurt changes lactose into lactic acid. Lactic acid is strong enough to precipitate milk protein into yogurt and will precipitate the proteins that the bacteria are living on and will kill most of the bacteria.

Reversing Coronary Artery Disease

Damage to the coronary arteries of the heart is reversible. Most by-pass surgery can be prevented if one aggressively tries to repair the damage. If one stops smoking and stops taking nicotine patches, while paying close attention to diet, exercise and medication, there is a very good chance that the arteries will be back to normal in three years. Total cholesterol should be under 150. LDL cholesterol (the bad cholesterol) should be below 60 and HDL cholesterol (the good cholesterol) should be above 45. The BMI (Body Mass Index) should be between 19 and 23. One should be walking at a rapid pace for 30 minutes a day or doing some equivalent exercise for 30 minutes a day. If one wants to repair damaged coronary arteries one has to do more than what one does to prevent damage. The numbers given are for repair.

Heart Attack

Five year olds don't get heart attacks but teenagers already do, and as they get older, they get more plaque and eventually the blood cannot get through, a little piece breaks off and goes to the brain – and that's called a stroke or a Transient Ischemic Attack (T.I.A.). T.I.A. is a stroke that lasts less than 24 hours. For example, a definite paralysis of the right arm for 5 hours. No matter what one tries to do one cannot move the arm. An hour later normal motion returns. What has happened is a broken bit of cholesterol plaque has gone through the artery to that part of the brain that serves the right arm. The initial blockage causes a spasm that shuts down a lot of blood flow but the spasm stops and blood flow returns to most of that part of the brain, and function returns.

If there is fat in the body, the body makes more cholesterol, which is deposited in the walls of the arteries, forming a flat cake (plaque) on the walls of the arteries. After a while the cake comes loose at one end and the other sticks to the wall. The artery is blocked, no blood flow and no oxygen gets to the heart muscle and one has a heart attack. If the artery is one of the three that go to the brain, one has a stroke.

A 60 year old man who had heart surgery was put on a low cholesterol diet which he followed strictly for three years and his heart had gotten much stronger. He then decided to have a party on a Thursday night where he had filet mignon, apple pie with ice cream, and all the foods he was not supposed to eat. On Saturday he went for his regular bi-monthly visit and had a blood draw. The blood results were quite good and nothing happened in the 3 days between the time he ended his diet and he had a blood test. Two days later he decided to go on a vacation. After being in Florida for 10 days where he ate all the foods he was not supposed to eat, he came back, and lo and behold, his cholesterol was sky high, and he was in pretty bad shape. He was back about one week when he had a heart attack and died, the price he paid for having gone off his diet.

By-pass Surgery

A man was in a reputable hospital for by-pass surgery to be performed the next day, when his private doctor came in to see him. The doctor looked at his chart and told him: "You don't need to have the surgery. If you have it and live the way you've been living, you will have to have by-pass surgery again in about 8 or 9 years." The patient was afraid of his surgeons, since one of them tried to blackmail him by saying: "If you don't have this operation, you are going to have to pay for all the time you've been in the hospital." That was $11,000. His private doctor reassured him that the insurance would pay for it whether he had the operation or not, and as a matter of fact, the insurance company would be happy to have him avoid the operation because it saves them a lot of money.

By 7 o'clock in the evening he got up his courage and, against the surgeon's advice, signed out. His private doctor then put him on a low cholesterol diet, an exercise program and got him off smoking. That was nine years ago and he did very well and is still sticking to the diet. He gets exercise every day and does not smoke. His children are very happy and proud of papa.

The mortality rate for by-pass surgery is about 5% – or one chance in twenty of dying from the surgery. Most people (80%) who have had by-pass surgery, have it repeated 8 or 9 years after the first one.

3. Cigarette Smoking

Cigarette Smoking Events

In 1946 at the Army Chemical Center in Maryland about twenty people were accidentally exposed to nerve gas. Nerve gas was being manufactured in a small, secret plant on the shores of the Chesapeake Bay. On the day of the accident one of the men running the plant accidentally turned the wrong valve on a tank, dumping 10 gallons of nerve gas into the nearby swamp and went on to make the next batch. The valve for emptying the tank into the swamp was right next to the valve for entering a batch of nerve gas into the tank. The worker was in impervious clothing and had oxygen supplied from an oxygen tank. He had no idea of the accident. It was a lovely spring day and a gentle breeze was blowing from the nerve gas plant to the chlorine manufacturing plant 2.5 miles away and a mile further on to US Highway 40. Sixteen physicians from the research laboratory rushed to the scene to treat those who were exposed and went on to US 40 to see if people driving by were being poisoned, i.e. if people were pulling over to the side of the highway a ½ mile away. Nobody was pulling over, so no one on the highway was getting significant exposure. No one at the chlorine plant died, but some were very sick.

After it was all over and the people involved were moved out of the area, one of the poisoned people pulled out a cigarette, lit it, took one puff and dropped to the ground in shock. Blood pressure 60/00, clammy and pale. He was given atropine and oxygen and he recovered. It was impressive what a little bit of nicotine could do.

The patient really wanted to smoke, so several days later he tried standing down wind 12 – 15 feet from someone who was smoking. This caused him intestinal cramps, feeling faint, and difficulty breathing. By three weeks he could stand downwind within a foot. A week later he could take a puff and a week after that he could smoke.

Nerve gas destroys the enzyme cholinesterase. Cholinesterase destroys acetylcholine. If cholinesterase is completely destroyed the acetylcholine will very rapidly accumulate and death follows. When small amounts of acetylcholine accumulate one gets a bowel movement, slowing of the heart, dimming of vision, etc. Once any cholinesterase is destroyed it takes the body a month to replace it.

What a way to stop smoking! One exposure and the individual can't smoke for a month. This gives time to get used to not smoking. Repeated exposure to small doses of nerve gas causes no permanent damage according to the U.S. Army data. Once a month exposures to small doses of some of the nerve gas could keep a person off cigarettes for a long time. Nerve gas is not commercially available.

One of the physicians doing work at the research center was difficult to wake up in the morning in time to get breakfast. One day a stick of juicy fruit chewing gum was slipped under his pillow. This gum has the odor of one of the nerve gases. About 30 seconds later, without opening his eyes, he reached for his gas mask, put it on, jumped out of bed and rushed out the door. As he left the room he realized that there were two people in the room without masks on. He came back to the room very angry but it was pointed out to him that he was out of bed in time for breakfast.

Cockroaches love nerve gas. One part of the laboratory was infested with cockroaches. Occasionally, a small dose of nerve gas was put in a flat Petri dish under the hood at night before leaving the laboratory. At the top of the hood there was a fan that exhausted air from the hood so that no one would get injured working with poisonous chemicals. A small opening was made at the bottom of the hood and roaches went into the hood, piled up dead around the Petri dish in a water drop pattern 6 – 7 roaches high where the air was coming in but only one roach high 5 – 6 inches from the Petri dish in the direction the air was flowing.

Cigarette Smoking and Cancer of the Lungs

Smoking is a major problem in the United States. In 1895 there was an article in the Journal of the American Medical Association about a woman who had a cancer of the lung. A cancer of the lung in a woman was so rare that it warranted an article. Now the commonest cause of death due to cancer in a woman is cancer of the lung. 99% of all cancers of the lung are due to cigarette smoking. Cancers of the breast are more common than cancers of the lung, but half of the women with cancer of the breast are cured. Only 4 – 5% of women with cancer of the lung are cured. A woman who smokes is 3 times as likely to get cancer of the lung than a man of the same age who smokes. The difference is probably due to the estrogen in a woman's body.

Every puff of cigarette smoke irreversibly damages the lungs by making the cells of the lung susceptible to being converted to cancer cells by irradiation from cosmic rays that are constantly hitting the earth from outer space. Some of these cosmic rays are more powerful than any of the rays that an X-ray machine can make.

A woman can smoke ½ a pack a day for ten years when she was young and then stop. Forty years later she comes down with lung cancer. She is surprised that she has cancer of the lung and says: "I can't see why I have cancer of the lung. I haven't smoked for forty years." The more one smokes the more cells become susceptible to becoming cancerous. The lungs never completely recover. Cancer of the lung is scattered all through the lung and is best picked up by a CT scan of the lung. Attempts to find lung cancer early by taking annual CT scans have not been successful in finding lung cancer early enough that it can be successfully treated. If one does a bronchoscopy and a biopsy of the lining of the tubes of the lungs of a cigarette smoker, the whole lining appears as if it is made up of cancer cells. The cure rate is very small.

The combination of inhaling tobacco and incidental inhalation of asbestos can cause a particular kind of cancer, a *mesothelioma*, which occurs in the lining of the chest wall. There is no treatment for a mesothelioma. A mesothelioma is not related to a cancer of the lung. Life expectancy is 5 years.

Cigarette Smoking and Damage of the Lungs

In addition to causing cancer of the lungs, cigarette smoking causes the cells in the lung to become so damaged that only small amounts of oxygen can be absorbed. This is more likely to occur than cancer. Smoking alters the cells in the lung so that they cannot reproduce nor be repaired, so the number of cells in the lung gradually disappears. The structure of the lung changes. After 30 or 40 years the individual has what is called COPD (Chronic Obstructive Pulmonary Disease) or emphysema. When this becomes severe enough, ordinary air no longer carries enough oxygen into the lungs and not enough carbon dioxide out to keep one alive. One will need an oxygen concentrator in the home with 100 feet of light-weight plastic tubing attached to a facial mask. This is enough to get to most places in the house and one can carry out minor chores, like fixing up meals, etc. To go outside of the house one needs to carry a tank of oxygen. There are tanks one wears on one's back like a backpack or an oxygen tank on a two-wheel carrier to take when out of the home. On the average this will give one an additional three years of life. On or about then, pneumonia will end one's life. When the COPD becomes bad then there are two options: one is the oxygen tank route. The other is to continue smoking and fade away.

When the lungs are damaged, carbon dioxide accumulates in the body every day. If the lungs are badly damaged not only can one not get enough oxygen in and one also can not get enough carbon dioxide out. When the carbon dioxide gets to a certain level it becomes a sedative and anesthetic. As the concentration gets higher and higher one becomes drowsier and drowsier until one stops breathing.

Cigarette Smoking and the Heart

It isn't cancer that causes most of the deaths from smoking, nor is it COPD. When it comes to stopping smoking some people recommend nicotine patches or nicotine gum. This does not make sense. It is the nicotine that causes damage to the arteries. Heart attacks, damaged heart muscle, strokes, ruptured blood vessels, and blood clots in damaged blood vessels are all related to nicotine usage. In the United States 442,000 die each year of smoking.

Cigarette Smoking and Pregnancy

Studies have shown that a mother's smoking during pregnancy causes the baby's I.Q. to be 10 points lower than it would be if the mother had not been smoking. An I.Q. loss of 10 means that 67% of the population will be more intelligent than the newborn. Nicotine causes the blood vessels in the placenta to go into spasm and this shuts down the blood flow. The brain is the fastest growing part of the embryo and hence the most sensitive to a lack of oxygen. Exposure to second hand cigarette smoke should also be avoided.

How to Stop Smoking

Cigarette smokers often claim they want to stop smoking but they just can't. What they really mean is that they want something that produces the effects of nicotine but is not so dangerous. When offered a way of really stopping they usually say: "Well, I would like to think about it."

One way to stop smoking is to make it uncomfortable if one does smoke. This can be done by giving one the need to move one's bowels if they inhale cigarette smoke. The muscles in the walls of the colon will contract when the receptor sites along the muscle are stimulated by a sufficient amount of acetylcholine, or nicotine, or a combination of the two. When stimulated, the muscles contract and move their contents to the rectum and anus. The drug donepezil (Aricept) is a cholinesterace inhibitor. That is, it stops the destruction of acetylcholine which means that acetylcholine will accumulate in the receptor sites along the muscle. If we now add a little nicotine from cigarette smoke, that might be just enough to cause the muscle to contract and cause a bowel movement.

Donepezil has a half-life of 72 hours but is not a very powerful cholinesterace inhibitor. Rivastigmine (Exelon) is also a cholinesterace inhibitor. It is much stronger than donepezil but it has a half- life of only 1½ hours. The suggested regimen for the cigarette smoker is 10 mg of donepezil at bed time and 1.5 mg of rivastigmine as the first thing on wakening in the morning. Rivastigmine should also be taken before lunch and before supper. The reason for rivastigmine as the first thing in the morning is that the regular cigarette smokers smoke a cigarette as soon as they wake up. On awakening, only donepezil is effective and if one smokes then, the urge to defecate is only moderate. When rivastigmine is active the effect is strong.

If the smoker has taken the Exelon and lights up during the next hour after awakening, he will feel the need to go to the bathroom within 30 seconds of lighting the cigarette. In 3 – 4 minutes the urge would be really urgent. If one forgets the morning dose of rivastigmine and lights a cigarette, one will still have an urge to defecate due to the donepezil, but one may be able to wait 10 or 15 minutes.

One time a patient who was taking Aricept and Exelon decided to give up smoking completely, but kept on taking Exelon and Aricept. Two weeks later a friend offered him a cigarette. He took two puffs, and had the sudden urge to defecate. The nearest bathroom was three floors up. He ran as fast as he could and just made it. He never forgot again.

4. Obesity

Obesity is dangerous. It brings out diabetes in people who would ordinarily be normal. A large number of people have inherited the gene for diabetes but it does not cause any trouble, or if it does, it occurs very late in life – age 70 or 80. But if one overeats and becomes fat the gene is activated. It goes into action – nobody knows why. The cells in the body become resistant to insulin and have trouble absorbing glucose. Glucose is the source of energy for the cells in the body. Without glucose they die. If they don't die they are sick and do not function properly.

Glucose, the sugar that is present in the blood, is no longer easily used. It takes extra insulin to get the glucose into the cells. The muscles need the glucose in order to get the energy for contracting but have trouble getting the glucose. At the same time that the extra insulin is helping the cells to get glucose in them, the extra insulin increases the appetite so the individual eats more. Now we have extra glucose and this gets converted to fat.

If children are eating more food than is needed, the food turns to fat. High calorie food like pizza, candies, ice cream, cookies, etc. cause children to become fat quickly. Physical energy uses up glucose and helps to prevent obesity. The excess glucose that goes with diabetes results in blindness, damaged kidneys, and hardening of the arteries.

It is important for children to exercise because if they don't, they gain weight and get fat and that leads to trouble.

The body has to make cholesterol. It is essential. Every single cell in the body has a membrane around it that has cholesterol in it. With all that extra confined cholesterol floating around, it is easy to deposit cholesterol where it is not needed. A rigid low fat diet can cause the body to make less cholesterol. One doesn't need the 200 mg/dl of cholesterol which most people have. One has to start watching cholesterol intake at about age 5.

Teenagers too often ignore a healthy diet, claiming: "All my friends and my parents have bacon and eggs for breakfast." Intelligent adults think: "It won't be me – I won't have a heart attack."

Obesity is a major problem in North America, Europe and most of the rest of the inhabited parts of the world. A lot of work is going into the search for a treatment with little promise on the horizon. A number of drugs and diets help a bit when people first start to follow them but after 6 months the progress diminishes or stops.

Analysis of Some Popular Programs for Losing Weight

There are very few controlled, randomized studies comparing one method with another. One such study was done in Boston at the Tufts New England Medical Center in 2004 and published in the Journal of the American Medical Association in January 5, 2005. It involved 160 people who were randomly assigned to one of 4 diets. 40 people to each diet.
After one year these were the results:

Diet	Average total loss in pounds in one year	No. of people who remained on the diet for one year
Atkins	10.6	21
Zone	13.2	26
Weight Watchers	10.8	26
Ornish	16.1	20

The weight lost did not amount to much. Although there was a great difference between the diets, there was virtually no difference in the amount of weight loss.

The characteristics for each of the diets are outlined below.

Atkins Diet

The Atkins Diet has been controversial for 40 years. It consists of eating fat and protein and as little carbohydrate as possible. This causes ketoacidosis which makes one feel sick.

There is no question that it causes weight loss. But very few people can stay on the diet for more than 3 years. They get tired of eating it and one day they try eating a doughnut or its equivalent. Nothing dramatic happens to them and they try it again and again, and soon they are off the diet and the weight rises back to where it used to be. There is no evidence that the diet decreases the chance of heart attack or stroke.

Barry Sears' "Zone" Diet

A person following the "Zone" diet tries to maintain a constant ratio of protein eaten to that of carbohydrate eaten at the same time. The ratio is 3 grams of protein to 4 grams of carbohydrate. However, protein from a meat source is more completely digested than that from a vegetable source. The program does not give any way of calculating how much vegetable protein is equal to a protein from a meat source.

The "Zone" book was copyrighted in 1995 and at that time the value of fish oil was already well recognized and yet the "Zone" still concentrated on the ratio of protein to carbohydrate while overlooking the value of fish oil. The amount of fat in the diet encourages an increase in cholesterol.

Insulin is an appetite stimulant. The higher the insulin is the higher one's appetite, the hungrier one is. A high sugar level is what one tries to avoid in people with diabetes. A high sugar level causes the pancreas to put out more insulin. The extra insulin is all right for normal people but it is bad for those with diabetes or borderline diabetes. The "Zone" Diet does not emphasize lowering insulin concentration.

The samples given by the "Zone" diet included hamburgers, bacon, peanuts, mayonnaise, mozzarella cheese but no other milk products. Cottage cheese was listed as a "protein block", yet the quantity is a mystery. There is only one example of a vegetarian protein, tofu. Tofu contains phytoestrogens which will enlarge a man's nipple and make it painful. It also has 8% fat. Peanut oil, which he recommends is highly atherogenic, that is, it causes hardening of the arteries, heart attacks and strokes. All vegetables contain proteins but he is not aware of it.

Ornish Diet

The Ornish Diet allows fish and fish oil only if you don't have coronary artery disease. This is a mistake since fish oil has been proven to be beneficial in preventing heart attacks and stroke. Most cardiologists recommend fish oil and fish if one has heart disease.

Ornish recommends staying away from all nuts which is also a mistake. Some nuts are very valuable. Gamma linolenic acid is an essential fatty acid since it cannot be made by the body and the body requires it to make myelin. Myelin is the covering around most of the nerves in the brain. Gamma linolenic acid is found in walnuts, Brazil nuts, and some meat products.

Most nuts (with the exception of walnuts and Brazil nuts) should be avoided because the fatty acids they contain are not good. Oils should be avoided with the exception of olive oil, which the Ornish diet is opposed to. Small amounts of olive oil, one teaspoon a day, will not do any harm.

A problem with the Ornish Diet is that it requires a lot of time in the preparation and cooking.

Weight Watchers Diet

Weight Watchers has two programs, one called the "Core Program" and the other the "Points Program".

The Core Program: One is given a list of approved Core Program foods that one can eat as much as one needs in order to feel satisfied. The program offers suggestions on how to determine when one is satisfied.
In addition to the approved foods, one has 35 points per week to eat items not on the approved list. There is a very wide selection on the non approved list including ice cream, alcoholic beverages, peanut butter, potato chips, etc.

The Point System: Points are assigned to all things eaten and one has an allotment per day. 650 items have points assigned. Whatever one wants to eat one has to add up the number of points that they require and limit oneself to only that amount of food on one day. The number of points per day varies from 43 for someone weighing 340 lbs to 30 for someone under 150 lbs. Items on the list include all kinds of meat but no items that have a large fat content. The program emphasizes exercise and also attending weekly meetings, discussing problems, and getting weighed.

Other Regimens

Frozen Foods

Companies put out packages of frozen food with the total number of calories on the package. They suggest eating only this product and the number of calories that one is supposed to eat. Others suggest that the main meal of the day should be only one of these products and calories should be around 600.

Adrenergic Drugs for Weight Loss

These are drugs like diethylpropion (Tenuate), methylphenidate (Ritalin), phentermine (Adipex), dextroamphetamine (Dexedrine). They are related to the chemicals epinephrine and norepinephrine, which the body makes and releases in order to control blood pressure. They all help losing weight. However, used steadily for 3 – 6 months, the body becomes used to them and one no longer loses weight. If one is tolerant to one of the drugs, one is partially tolerant to all. They all have the same basic mechanism. Combining the medications can be dangerous.

Lipase Inhibitor

Orlistat (Xenical) is a lipase inhibitor. It stops the absorption of fat from the intestine. In order to be absorbed, a fat must be broken apart into fatty acids. Orlistat prevents this, and the fat goes through the intestine and comes out in the stool untouched. This makes the stool greasy, but most people can put up with it. Using orlistat, a group of 2,800 people with diabetes lost an average of 13.4 pounds a year and regained ½ of that by 4 years.

Neurotransmitter Reuptake Inhibitors

The only one used for obesity is sibutramine (Meridia). It inhibits the reuptake of serotonin, norepinephrine and dopamine at nerve endings and this is the same set of transmitters that venlafaxine (Effexor), a very effective antidepressant, inhibits. On a year long study of the effects of sibutramine, the patients on the placebo (a pill that looks and tastes like the active one but has no medication in it) lost 3.5 lbs, and those taking 10 mg of sibutramine a day lost 9.8 lbs.

Exercise

A very important part of weight loss is exercise. Some exercise is essential. It is very difficult to lose weight or to prevent gaining weight without getting some exercise. The minimum is the equivalent of walking a mile a day. More exercise will be helpful.

A Stringent Cholesterol Lowering Diet

This diet has three aims:

1. To markedly decrease the intake of animal fats, except for fish oil.
2. To decrease the intake of vegetable oil.
3. To limit the total amount of cholesterol ingested.

Aim 1 (Low animal fat)

Except for the fat in fish (fish oil), the total amount of fat in the diet should be between 5 and 8 grams (gm) per day. The limit is relaxed to 13 to eat 100 gm of chicken (3 oz) once a week but this should be lean chicken and should not include chicken skin. Whole milk has the same kind of fat in it as does steak (both milk and steak come from cattle). Hence, no whole milk, no cream, no butter and no regular cheese. However, skim milk or reconstituted powdered milk is all right.
Fish oil contains a special type of fat composed of omega 3 fatty acids which are beneficial.

Aim 2 (Low vegetable oil)

Vegetable oils, which are fats, must be sharply restricted. Cocoa is ok, but chocolate is not. Chocolate is composed of equal parts of cocoa and cocoa butter.

Aim 3 (Low cholesterol content)

The only cholesterol in the diet should come from sea foods.

Type of Food	Permitted	Forbidden
Beverages	Orange juice (0.03%)*, Tomato juice (0.1%), All fruit and vegetable juices, Coffee without: cream, non-dairy creamer or whole milk, Tea, Carbonated beverages, Wine (6 oz) or beer (12 oz) or Whiskey (1 oz)**	Coconut milk (25%)* More than an average of one drink per day
Dairy Products	Skim milk or non-fat milk (0.1%)*, Reconstituted powdered milk (0.2%), Non-fat yogurt (0.5%), Non-fat frozen yogurt (0.5%), Sherbet (1.2%), Non-fat cottage cheese (0.5%), Non-fat cream cheese, Non-fat cheese cake, Fat-Free cheese	Butter (81%)*, Cream (21%), Buttermilk (0.9%), Whole milk (3.7%), 2% low-fat milk, Sour cream (20%), Ice cream (10 – 16%), Ice milk (5%), Condensed or evaporated milk (10%), Creamed cottage cheese (4.7%), Regular cheese (30%), Skim milk cheese (4.7%), Cream cheese (37%), Non-dairy creamer (35%), Whipped topping (25%)
Breads, Cereals, and Grain Products	Bakery made bagel (0.5%)*, Italian bread (1%), French bread (1%), Sourdough bread (1.7%), English muffin (2%), Fat-free sandwich buns,	Supermarket bagel (3 – 5%)*, Rye (3.6%), Pumpernickel (2.4%), Pita Bread (4%), Croissants (24%), Cornbread (7%),

* (0.0%) after an item indicates its fat content

** Quantities per day

Type of Food	Permitted	Forbidden
Breads, Cereals, and Grain Products (cont'd)	Light bread (white, whole wheat, rye, or mixed) (2%)*, Fat-free saltines (Premium), Oatmeal (1%), Cream of wheat (0.2%), Fat-free breakfast cereals, Corn flakes, Corn Chex (0.3%), Grape nuts, Special K (0.3%), Puffed Rice (0.0%), Rice Chex (0.1%), Wheaties (1.7%), Shredded wheat (2%), Spaghetti, Macaroni (0.5%), Pasta (0.2%), Pretzels (1.1%), Popcorn (5%) (no butter), Sweet corn (1%) (Field corn (4%)), Pancakes (Aunt Jemima, ½ the usual olive oil) (1.1%), Low Fat Tofu	Muffins (11%)*, Biscuits (17%), Hamburger bun (5 – 6%), White or whole wheat bread (4%), Corn chips (40%), Tortillas (25%), Ritz crackers (29%), Granola (17%), Heartland (15%), Nutri- Grain (13%), 100% Bran (5%), Cheerios (6%), Raisin Bran (2.4%), Wheat germ (10%)
Fruits and Vegetables	Any fruit (fresh, canned, frozen or juiced), Most vegetables (raw, baked, or boiled), Lentils (0.2%)*, Potato (0.1%), Yam (0.2%), Peas (0.4%), Lima beans (0.5%), Green beans (0.2%), Broccoli (0.3%), Potato Chips cooked in Olean, French Fries cooked in Olean	Creamed or fried vegetables, French fried potatoes (8 – 14%)*, Hash-browned potatoes (12%), Potato chips (40%), Avocados (16%), Vegetable oils (100%)

Type of Food	Permitted	Forbidden
Fish, Poultry, and Meat	All ocean raised fish (Only they contain omega 3 fatty acid, the desirable fatty acid),*** Salmon (13 – 15%)*, Mackerel (12%), Shad (10%), Canned sardines in water (12%), Striped bass (3%), Bluefish (3%), Halibut (1.2%), Tuna (4%), Swordfish (4%), Canned tuna in water (0.9%), Flounder (0.8%), Cod (0.3%), Crab (1.9%), Scallops (0.2%), Shrimp (0.8%) – no more than 3 oz. per week (high cholesterol)**** Chicken – white meat (5%), Chicken – dark meat (7%), Turkey – the same as chicken, Egg whites (0.03%), Egg beaters (0.0%), Lean, red meat, when permitted – separable fat must be removed,	Chicken skin (29%)*, Bologna (27%), Salami (38%), Hamburger (20%), Frankfurters (27%)*, Steak with fat (43%), Bacon (cooked, drained) (52%), Liver (11%), Heart (29%), Pork chops (15%), Pancreas (sweet bread) (20%), Most gravies, Lobster (1.9%) (high cholesterol), Oyster (1.8%) (high cholesterol), Whole eggs (12%), Egg yolk (31%)

*** The percent fat figures are for raw fish. Broiled and baked fishes are generally basted with butter while being cooked. Baked flounder contains 8% fat as compared to 0.8% for the raw fish. This means 7.2% butter fat in baked flounder. Broiled and basted bluefish contains 5.4 % fat versus 3% raw. For halibut it is 7% versus 1.2% and for swordfish 6% versus 4%. Poaching or steaming or microwaving does not add butter fat. *When asking for fish in a restaurant, ask for fish broiled or baked "dry".*

**** Three large shrimp or 5 – 7 medium shrimp (3 inches long) weigh 100 gms.

Type of Food	Permitted	Forbidden
Fish, Poultry, and Meat (cont'd)	Ham (9%)*, Steak (10%), Leg of lamb (8%)	
Soup	Clear broth, consomme, bouillon, Fat free vegetable soup, Pritikin fat free soups Packaged dehydrated soups, only if they are not creamy	Pea soup made with water Cream of mushroom (Milk)
Desserts and Sweets	Angel Food Cake, Jello, Non-fat cakes, cookies and pastries, Puddings made with skim milk, Marshmallows (0%), Jelly beans, Jam, Jelly, Honey, Syrup, Walnuts (59%; 12% is gamma linolenic), Brazil Nuts (67%; 46% is gamma linolenic)	Regular cakes, pies and cookies, Devil's food cake (19%), Apple pie (10 – 16%), Oatmeal cookies (15%), Brownies (31%), Danish pastries (23%), Doughnuts (18 – 26%), Chocolate candy, Coconut (39%), Peanuts (49%) (cause heart attacks in monkeys), Cashews (46%)
Miscellaneous	Salt, Pepper, Spices, Herbs, Pickles (0.2%), Non-fat salad dressings: Ranch, Russian, Italian, etc. ***** Non-fat Miracle Whip Cocoa, Chocolate Syrup	Pizza, All other salad dressings, All oil including olive oil, Mayonnaise, Coconut oil is especially bad

***** Read the labeling of ingredients carefully. Some food companies are dishonest and label a salad dressing as "Fat Free", when it does contain fat in the form of soybean oil.

Olive oil is better than butter fat but no olive oil is better yet. If you need fat, use olive oil.

Cholesterol

The average U.S. diet contains 750 mg of cholesterol per day. The average for South East Asia is 30 mg/day. Current recommendations are under 300 mg/day. No vegetables, vegetable oils, or nuts contain any cholesterol.

Food	Cholesterol (mg/100gm)
Salmon	35
Cod, Halibut, Tuna	50-60
Sardines	120
Scallops	35
Crab	100
Shrimp	150
Lobster	200
Oysters	230
Caviar	280
Red meat (fat removed)	85
Liver	285
Sweetbreads	303
Poultry (without skin)	80
Chicken Liver	486
Chicken Gizzard	123
Whole Milk	13
Skimmed Milk	1.6
Reconst. Powder Milk	1.6
Low Fat Yogurt	4.6
Cheese	70
Imitation cheese	3
Cottage Cheese	3
Ice Cream	40
Ice Milk	14
Butter	240
Egg Yolk	1480

XII
Death

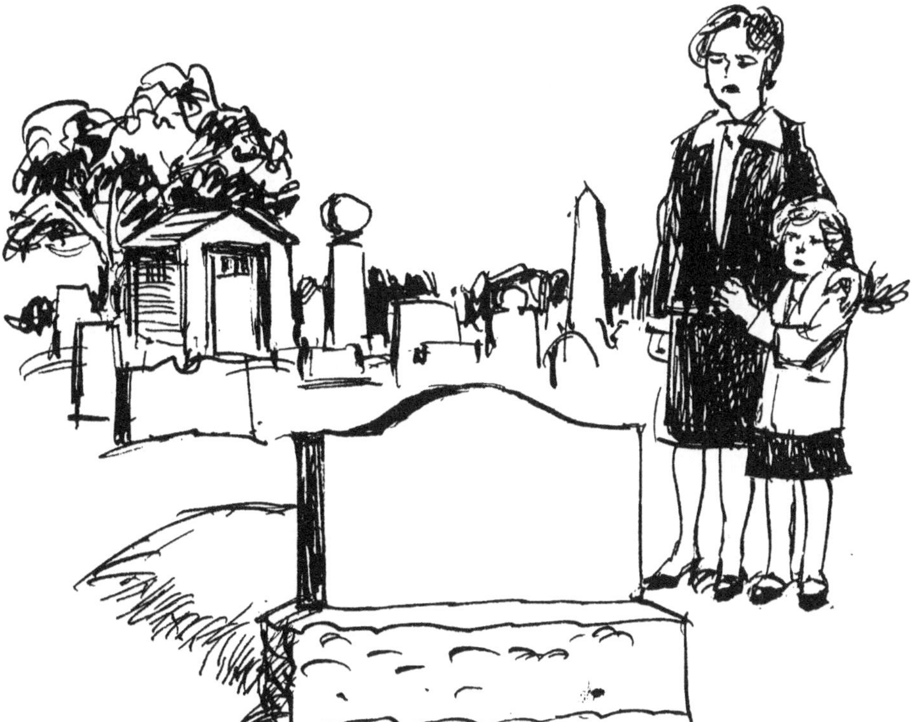

Death

From the moment of birth one instinctively tries to avoid danger and illness – to delay the inevitable – death. Overindulgence in childhood takes on a lifetime trend which speeds the demise of people who overeat, eat the wrong foods, smoke, drink too much alcohol, etc.

Life is a temporary condition. People who behave as though life is "forever" miss deadlines and postpone responsibilities. The "instant" person attends to responsibilities and when he says he'll do something, he does it, respecting others as well as his own mortality.

Dying creates a vacancy which triggers a chain reaction. It's like a piece falling off a mobile, where all remaining pieces must be shifted to adjust to the new balance. Imagining the future while alive prolongs life in one's imagination.

Children whose parents do not have a Living Will may be forced to make life and death decisions for their parents, which potentially can leave a scar of guilt.

Parents who don't leave a Will, control their children's lives when they assign two executors to their Will and the executors don't get along, or if they leave more to one child, or eliminate one child from their Will, causing acrimony among the siblings and the inheritance is spent on attorneys. Parents have done a wonderful job if their children remain on speaking terms with each other their entire lives.

Although tears are associated with sorrow and pain, to a great degree tears are an expression of rage. In the case of losing someone, there is a component of anger at having suffered the loss. The close survivors, with few exceptions, experience guilt, regardless of whether the guilt is based on fact. While speaking well of the deceased, it is also helpful to point to the survivors that they were helpful to the deceased in his/her lifetime. At a time of bereavement, when a person is in touch with his deep feelings, a clear recognition of the need for exchange of positive feelings is crystallized.

Often, it is not until a loved one expires that remorse for not having expressed positive feelings towards him in his lifetime, gnaws at his family and friends. This is also demonstrated by the practice of only posthumously (and sometimes never) bestowing glowing recognition on great men and women of history.

Too often adults remember their childhood as "abusive" and proceed to retaliate against their aged parents by neglecting or criticizing them when the parents are near the end of their lives. All parents make mistakes, yet they gave their children the greatest gift of all – life! The young often lack understanding that the old, too, want to live, unless depression or incurable painful illness has set in. Looking in the mirror at every age takes adjustment. However, when a person ages, his eyesight deteriorates as well, and when looking in the mirror he sees himself looking young.

The hypochondriac believes that he faces imminent death every day of his life, an all-encompassing, burdensome emotional problem. The hypochondriac neglects to ask the physician that last question in order to be fully reassured, knowing full well that there will still be another question, and yet another question and the reassurance will last only moments. Hypochondriacs die too, so their symptoms and complaints cannot be disregarded.

Very little in life is an emergency. When one behaves as though something is an emergency when it is not, it can lead to all kinds of trouble. Decisions made in great haste when there is no urgency are often mistakes that are later regretted. In a true emergency, the medical and/or legal profession must evaluate the symptoms.

A person who is continually miserable induces in others the urge to get him out of their sight or altogether put him out of his misery and symbolically "kill" him off.

A suicidal person wants to kill someone else and instead kills himself. In the case of a suicide bomber, he kills himself and kills others at the same time, while trying to make it appear as a "selfless act".

Should soldiers who abused prisoners and humiliated them sexually be punished? A 22 year old American reservist in the Abu Ghraib prison in Iraq was quoted as saying that soldiers had taken pictures of the naked pyramid of detainees because "it looked funny". She herself was photographed holding a naked detainee by a leash, while confessing that she stepped on some of the detainees and made them crawl on the wet floor for four hours. Surely her parents had done something drastically wrong with her upbringing, most likely caused by overindulgence throughout her childhood!!! The torture inflicted on the detainees showed a lack of empathy. Her parents or whoever brought her up should be punished – so that once and for all, future attention will be paid to the dangers of overindulging children!!

The owners of a dog who taught him to kill, were jailed once he killed a neighbor. Yet parents whose offspring kill are legally innocent. Surely, these parents did something wrong in bringing up killers. Taking this further, should an army veteran, having been taught to kill, once discharged committing murder, be considered innocent? The dog may have been taught to kill, but so was the draftee.

A teenager who invited the girl next door to watch T.V. and ended up killing her and cutting off her legs, once caught and apprehended, his attorney revealed that his client was "scared". Scared? What was the girl who was stabbed, killed and had her legs cut off? A person who callously commits a crime unaware of the victim's fear and pain, and who only betrays panic and fear when he himself is on the witness stand, lacks empathy and is the product of overgratification growing up. Parents, at any age, should be held emotionally and legally accountable for their children's crimes.

Recently an 80 year old clansman was sentenced to a 16 year prison term. It is never too late to punish a person who has been found guilty of committing a crime.

A front page photograph of a blinded soldier viewed by those with eyesight, brings home the horror of war. Closing one's eyes is relaxing, while being blind for the rest of one's life breeds desperation and depression. It's the death of eyesight!

Summary

Overindulged children grow up into pathologically jealous deceptive adults deserving the academy award for convincing everyone how wonderful, sweet and honest they are, while permanently dependent on a host. Strict discipline is practiced by responsible parents, while overindulgence is practiced by short sighted parents.

Children subjected to constant adulation grow up with unrealistic expectations, and an inability to deal with all thoughts and feelings, while hiding under the blanket of life using food, alcohol and cigarettes to flush out negative thoughts.

A child who is permitted to disregard his parents' commands will eventually write his own dictionary where "No" will be defined as "Yes", "Now" will be "Later", "Stop" will be "Continue", the words "Hurry up" will mean "Slow down", "Be punctual" will mean "Any time is okay".

The self indulgent parent when saying "no" to himself, then, in a moment of weakness gives in, sets a bad example for his children. The parent who eats too much, the wrong foods, drinks too much alcohol, smokes, is sexually perverse, and sets the alarm but remains in bed, sends the message: "Do as I say, not as I do".

Rarely heeding the warning that over-gratification can create a non-functioning adult with unreasonable expectations, the child raised by over-indulgent parents never ventures out of the "womb". The indulgent parent, while feeling that he is doing his best for his child, actually destroys the child's emotional and physical muscles, while the disciplined child grows up knowing boundaries between mine and yours and between truth and lies. Over-gratification is lethal, which is difficult for many parents to understand and believe, since it seems that being sweet, nice, kind, gentle and giving to the child from day one creates a happy and successful adult. Well, Surprise! The child will grow up unable to cope with life, where frustration will be an unfamiliar and overwhelming experience. Because of the rare times the parent was strict, such occasions will be recalled as parental abuse, while the parent who metes out constant discipline will toughen his child, enabling him to cope with life.

Index

(**Hint for the user**: Page numbers with 'f' or 'ff' refer to the following page(s) as well, which usually indicates a more detailed reference to the topic.)

Around the Subject

The Authors

Dr. Ruth Velikovsky Sharon learned at the desk of her distinguished father, Dr. Immanuel Velikovsky, a prominent psychiatrist and eminent man of science whose genius engaged even the mind of his friend and contemporary, Albert Einstein.

Dr. Sharon received a B.A and M.A. degrees from New York University and a Ph.D. from the Union Institute and University. She is a graduate of the Center for Modern Psychoanalytic Studies and a certified psychoanalyst.

Among Dr. Sharon's works are two books about her father: "The Glory and the Torment", and "The Truth Behind the Torment", which chronicles the controversy surrounding her father's extraordinary scientific theories. A book about a new dream theory: "Shame on You – You Were in my Dream" and co-author of the popular book "I Refuse to Raise a Brat".

Dr. John Cathro Seed was an undergraduate at Princeton University, and received his medical degree from Harvard University in 1945. His internship was at the Massachusetts General Hospital. In the first month of internship he and a colleague were the first to cure bacterial endocarditis, an infection of valves of the heart.

He was awarded the Pro Ecclesia et Pontifice by Pope John XXIII in 1962 for building Cavalry Hospital for dying cancer patients.

Dr. John Seed taught computer applications in medicine at Princeton University 1963 – 1985. Visiting Lecturer at Cornell Medical College; primary care physician at Martin Luther King Health Center 1966 – 1980 and Albert Einstein College of Medicine 1967 – 1983. Solo practice 1980 – present in Princeton. Attending physician at the University Medical Center at Princeton 1982 – present.

The First Blood Bank in The United States

Contributed by Randolph Seed, M.D.

In March of 1937, the first blood bank in the United States was opened at Cook County Hospital, in Chicago, Illinois. The announcement was posted on the door of Dr. Lindon Seed – Director of the Transfusion Service. It was established by Dr. Bernard Fantus with the help of Dr. Lindon Seed (father of John and Randolph Seed), who was the director of the transfusion services at Cook County Hospital.

At that time, all blood transfusions were direct transfusions from living donors to the patients. Dr. Lindon Seed, who had been trained in the early 20s at the Mayo Clinic, had rotated on the pernicious anemia service, which, at that time, had only a direct transfusion as the treatment for the disease. As a surgeon at Cook County Hospital, the same system was the only way to correct major blood loss from surgery and trauma and disease.

Dr. Bernard Fantus was a professor of therapeutics at the University of Illinois Medical School. He had been referred to Dr. Lindon Seed because he wanted to establish a "Blood Preservation Laboratory". Dr. Fantus had been studying the Soviet Union's "Blood Depot", which had been established since the early 1930's. By 1936, the USSR had more than 500 depots and they used selected cadaver blood for their source.

Dr. Fantus worked on improving the preservation of blood. He was referred to Dr. Lindon Seed who was the head of the transfusion service to start such a system. Because Dr. Lindon Seed had spent six months on the pernicious anemia service at the Mayo Clinic, he knew he could get live donors for the proposed "blood preservation laboratory" that Dr. Fantus wanted to set up.

Dr. Lindon Seed did not want to use Cook County cadavers for the blood source since he used to practice surgical operations in the Cook County Morgue Sunday mornings (after the Saturday night shootings) and had a very negative attitude towards the safety of such blood.

Dr. Lindon Seed's secretary of the transfusion service heard the discussions and she said: "It sounds like a bank – putting in deposits". She is unheralded as the one who suggested the idea for the name – certainly an improvement over "Blood Preservation Laboratory". Though Cook County Hospital likes to claim it was the first blood bank in the world, it was only the first in the U.S.

Dr. Fantus was not an active clinician using blood. Dr. Lindon Seed was a surgeon and in need of readily available blood for transfusions. Their combined interests and efforts worked. It rapidly became accepted and effective at Cook County Hospital. Yet even in the first year or two, some doctors thought direct transfusion was better. In the published report of the November 9, 1938 Scientific Meeting of the Chicago Medical society, Dr E. H. Fell stated: "It is believed that fresh blood transfusion is and will continue to be the transfusion of choice". This was 20 months after the founding of the Blood Bank.

Dr. Bernard Fantus was the motivating force and academician. Dr. Lindon Seed was the clinician and practical surgeon and as the Director of the Transfusion Service could make it medically acceptable (there were resistors on the Medical Staff at Cook County) and a beneficial advance. Each had many other interests and I suspect neither thought it was any more than another of multiple steps towards improved patient outcome and lower mortality rates.

Dr. Fantus died in April, 1940 and never saw the widespread benefits of his efforts. Dr. Lindon Seed died in March of 1979 and had no long-term involvement in blood banks. He was a surgeon and this had solved one of surgery's major clinical problems. By 1942 he was in the US Army. He was Chief Surgeon of a 3000 bed general hospital in Southern England, which had the lowest mortality rate of any such hospital during World War II. When he returned after W.W. II, he started the first private radioactive isotope lab in 1946, primarily for diagnosing and treating thyroid diseases. He did this, in part, because while he was gone, his entire practice as a thyroid surgeon had been taken over by the surgeons of the area that did not go to war and he had to re-establish his practice and an income to support his family. Nevertheless he did do 9000 thyroidectomies in his career. He probably was the only general surgeon to be president of the Society of Nuclear Medicine, which now has 16,000 members. He also became president of the American Thyroid Association, an elite group of about 300 thyroidologists.

Dr. Randolph Seed was accepted as undergraduate at Harvard College at age 16. He was the only person ever drafted out of a medical school class of the University of Chicago. While in the Army he broke the record of the Army Division of Intelligence and Athletic Performance.

During his surgical internship, he decided to get a Ph.D. in Biochemistry and his thesis was published in the National Academy of Science and communicated by Frits Lippman (Nobel Laureate). It, among other observations, was one of the first to demonstrate long lived m-RNA in mammalian cells, and therefore negated the general concept that m-RNA turnover was the final common rate-limiting step in cellular control. This was in the early stages of what is now Molecular Biology.

He finished his training at Northwestern Memorial Hospital (as it is now called) as Chief Surgical Resident in 1967. During the next 30 some years, he was: Chief Surgeon at Grant Hospital, President University of Chicago Biological Sciences Alumni Association, President Chicago Unit American Cancer Society, Board of Trustees, Chicago Medical Society, Board of Directors, Interqual.

In addition to over 70 publications of medical articles, he appeared in the Guinness Book of World Records for stair-climbing (100 flight record set in 1972 and vertical mile record – 500 flights set in 1970).

He belonged to the National Ski Patrol for about 20 years, ran many marathons (including Boston), ran four fifty mile ultra marathons, and the Western States 100 Mile Endurance Run over the Sierra Nevada mountains. The 100 mile race has a 17,000 vertical foot climb in the canyons and 22,000 feet down.

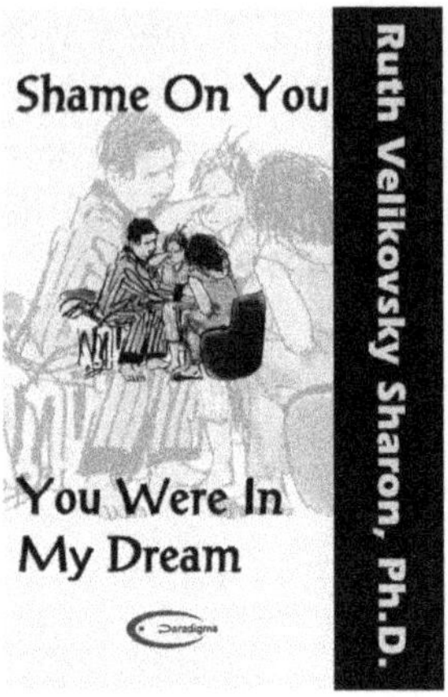

Shame on You – You Were in My Dream

by Ruth Velikovsky Sharon, Ph.D.

ISBN 978-1-906833-01-5

Finally a new and easy guide to the understanding of dreams, which really makes sense! Ruth Velikovsky Sharon, PhD has developed a completely new understanding of the nature of dreams, which is fascinating because of its simplicity and its practical orientation.
In her book, Dr. Sharon describes the way that parents can be of help vis a vis dreams. She includes chapters on manipulation in dreams, dream catchers and other gadgets and the environment and dreams.

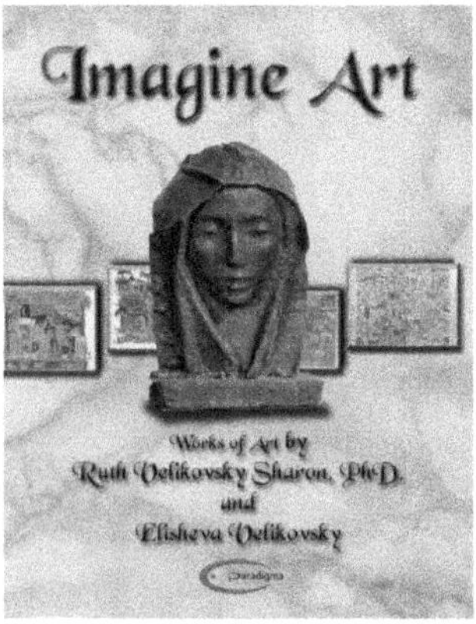

Imagine Art

**Works of Art by
Ruth Velikovsky Sharon, Ph.D.
and Elisheva Velikovsky**

ISBN 978-1-906833-02-2

The name of Velikovsky is mainly known from the scientific and historical discoveries of Dr. Immanuel Velikovsky.
Far less known is the artistic dimension in the Velikovsky family, mainly expressed by Elisheva (or "Elis") Velikovsky and Ruth Velikovsky Sharon, PhD., the wife and daughter of Immanuel Velikovsky. For everyone interested in and fond of visual and plastic arts this booklet will give an exhaustive overview of the remarkable range of the works of these two artists.

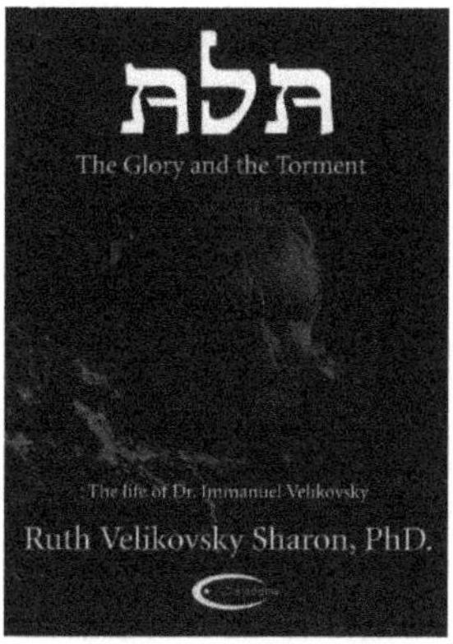

ABA – The Glory and the Torment

by Ruth Velikovsky Sharon, Ph.D.

ISBN 978-1-906833-20-6

In this book you get to know Immanuel Velikovsky as a person. His daughter Ruth describes his childhood, his family environment and his eventful life.

Using plenty of background information, numerous anecdotes and many photographs she makes us familiar with her father, but also shows the personal dimension of the devastating campaign he encountered to in the last decades of his life.

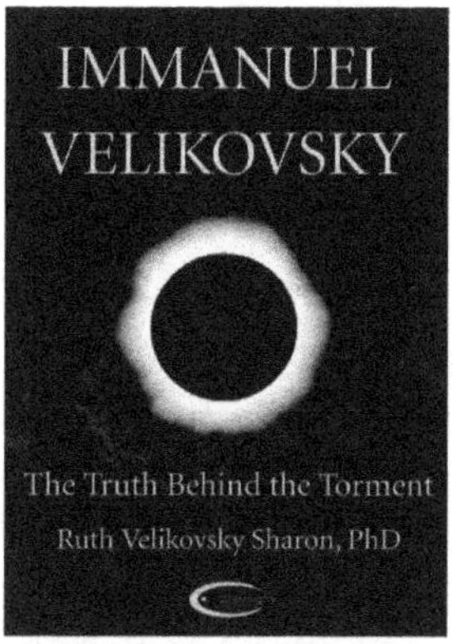

The Truth Behind the Torment

by Ruth Velikovsky Sharon, Ph.D.

ISBN 978-1-906833-21-3

In this supplement to her father's biography, Ruth Velikovsky Sharon, PhD. depicts the true facts about the campaign against him.

She publishes revealing letters in full length, that show the true nature of the undeserving - unscientific - treatment of Velikovsky by the scientific establishment, a treatment that appears rather medieval than enlightened.

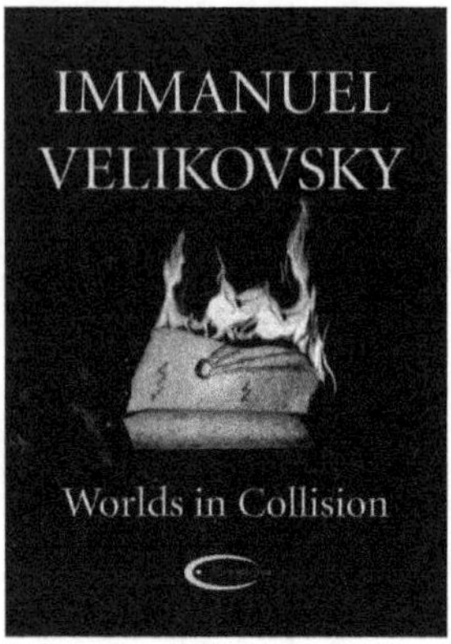

Worlds in Collision

by Immanuel Velikovsky

ISBN 978-1-906833-11-4

With this book Immanuel Velikovsky first presented the revolutionary results of his 10-year-long interdisciplinary research to the public - and caused an uproar that is still going on today.
Worlds in Collision - written in a brilliant, easily understandable and entertaining style and full to the brim with precise information - can be considered one of the most important and most challenging books in the history of science. Not without reason was this book found open on Einstein's desk after his death.

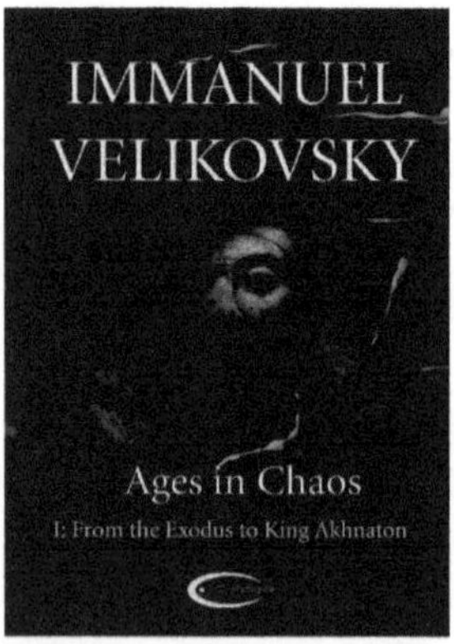

Ages in Chaos

by Immanuel Velikovsky

ISBN 978-1-906833-13-8

This is the first volume of the series *Ages in Chaos*, which undertakes a reconstruction of the history of antiquity.
With utmost precision and the exciting style of a presentation that's typical for him Immanuel Velikovsky shows what nobody would consider possible: In the conventional history of Egypt – and therefore also of many neighboring cultures – a span of 600 years is described, which has never happened! This assertion is as unbelievable and outrageous as the assertions in *Worlds in Collision* or *Earth in Upheaval*. But in the end you do not only wonder how conventional historiography has come into existence, but why it is still taught and published.

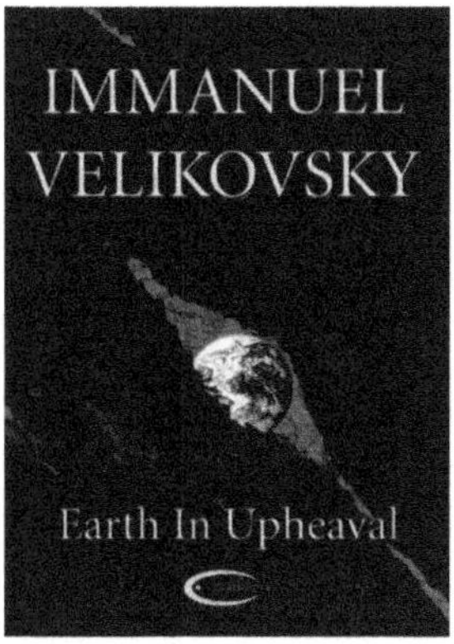

Earth in Upheaval

by Immanuel Velikovsky

ISBN 978-1-906833-12-1

After the publication of *Worlds in Collision* Immanuel Velikovsky was confronted with the argument that in the shape of the earth and in the flora and fauna there are no traces of the natural catastrophes he had described. Therefore a few years later he published *Earth in Upheaval* which not only supports the historical documents by very impressive geological and paleontological material, but even arrives at the same conclusions just based on the testimony of stones and bones.

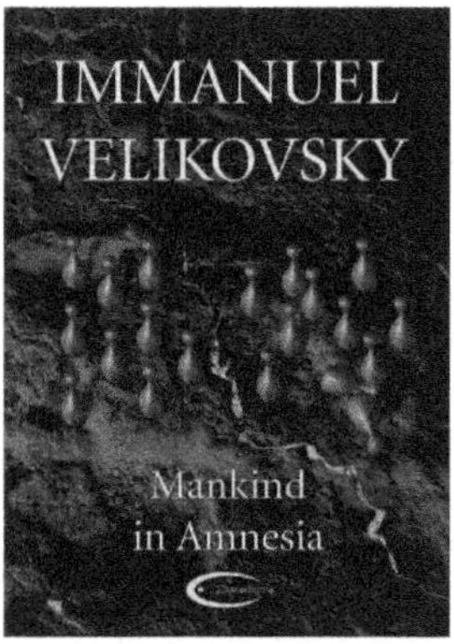

Mankind in Amnesia

by Immanuel Velikovsky

ISBN 978-1-906833-16-9

Immanuel Velikovsky called this book the "fulfillment of his oath of Hippocrates – to serve humanity." In this book he returns to his roots as a psychologist and psychoanalytical therapist, yet not with a single person as his patient but with humanity as a whole. After an extremely revealing overview of the foundations of the various psychoanalytical systems he takes the step into crowd psychology and reopens the case of *Worlds in Collision* from a totally different point of view: a psychoanalytical case study. This way he shows that the blatant reactions to his theories (which are still going on today) have not been surprising but actually inevitable from a psychological perspective.

www.ingramcontent.com/pod-product-compliance
Lightning Source LLC
Chambersburg PA
CBHW022132080426
42734CB00006B/333
* 9 7 8 1 9 0 6 8 3 3 0 0 8 *